365 ways to RELAX mind, body & soul

BARBARA L. HELLER

North Adams, Massachusetts

The mission of Storey Publishing is to serve our customers by publishing practical information that encourages personal independence in harmony with the environment.

Edited by Deborah Balmuth and Karen Levy
Cover and text design by Carol Jessop
Book layout by Susan Bernier
Production assistance by Deb Daly

Printed in the United States by Command Web
10 9 8 7 6 5 4 3

Library of Congress Cataloging-in-Publication Data

Heller, Barbara L.
365 ways to relax mind, body & soul / Barbara L. Heller.
p. cm.
ISBN 1-58017-332-2 (alk. paper)
1. Stress management. I. Title: three hundred and sixty five ways to relax mind, body & soul. II. Title.
RA785 .H45 2000
155.9'042--dc21 00-058795

Dedication

To my husband, Alan

Acknowledgments

My deep appreciation to my friend and writing companion extraordinaire, Paula Kephart, for your invaluable help and generosity.

Heartfelt thanks to my wonderful circle of support: Phyllis Heller, Barbara Ruchames, Bob Ruchames, Suzanne Massa, Irene Zahava, Tess Taft, and Zach Rosen for all your suggestions — and reminders to me to relax. Your friendship contributes enormously to the quality of my life.

I am also indebted to all those who trustingly share with me your personal struggles and triumphs. My life is richer for the experience.

A special thanks to my editors at Storey, Deborah Balmuth and Karen Levy, for the opportunity to write this book, and for your guidance and support.

My gratitude to my fantastic family: Thank you, Alan, for your sparkly eyed encouragement, your relaxed reading of the morning "rushes," and your helpful comments delivered with my morning coffee. Thanks for sharing my life.

And to Rebecca: Although parenting is not always relaxing, it is always gratifying because of the incredible person you are. Thanks for your encouragement, inspiration, thoughtfulness, and generous spirit.

Introduction

Are you stressed-out from juggling work, family, and personal activities? Feeling frazzled by excessive demands and information overload? If so, you are not alone. More than 20 million Americans suffer from stress-related illnesses. Many more are simply tired from the frenzied pace of modern life.

As a psychotherapist and educator for the past two decades, I have listened to clients, students, colleagues, and friends bemoan their increasing levels of stress, illness, and tension. And, of course, I have experienced my own challenges and anxieties. I have discovered that what we have in common is the need to develop better ways to respond to tension, loss, and frustration. We need to make more graceful transitions between our various roles and responsibilities, find new ways to wind down and replenish ourselves, and learn how to lighten up and appreciate our daily lives!

Most of us have not been taught how to relax. But relaxation is an acquired skill — one that you can learn. True relaxation creates a calm center to return to after stressful events and helps you feel renewed any time of the day. Relaxation also provides a peaceful counterpoint to positive stimulation. Releasing tension improves your immunity and heightens your creativity, effectiveness, intuition, and joy.

The benefits of relaxation are cumulative. Today, the gains may seem small, but, over time, you will be repaid with great riches. As you learn how to relax, you'll stop focusing primarily on your destination and you'll more fully enjoy the steps you take on your daily journey. The ripples will be far-reaching, affecting your family, workplace, and larger community. Relaxation will help you thrive, not just survive.

This little book offers you a broad range of relaxation techniques and soothing remedies and recipes. Many of the simple, practical tips you can try right now. Others require some planning and aim to create long-term solutions to stress. Start by choosing a couple of tips and incorporating them into your usual routine for five minutes a day. Build on your success. In the end, you will gain a healthier body, a calmer mind, and a more peaceful spirit.

Barbara L. Heller, M.S.W.

Express Your Creativity

All you need is a "little kid" coloring book with old favorite cartoon characters, an extra large box of crayons, and no artistic standards. And don't be afraid to color outside the lines!

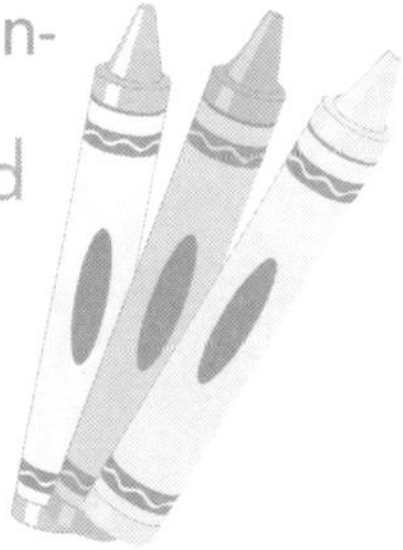

Clean Out the Clutter

Mental clutter may keep you from falling asleep, but physical clutter can affect you as well. Take some time this week to clean up the piles of clothes, stacks of magazines, or numerous knick-knacks that are cluttering your bedroom. A simplified environment serves as a natural sedative.

Go Retro

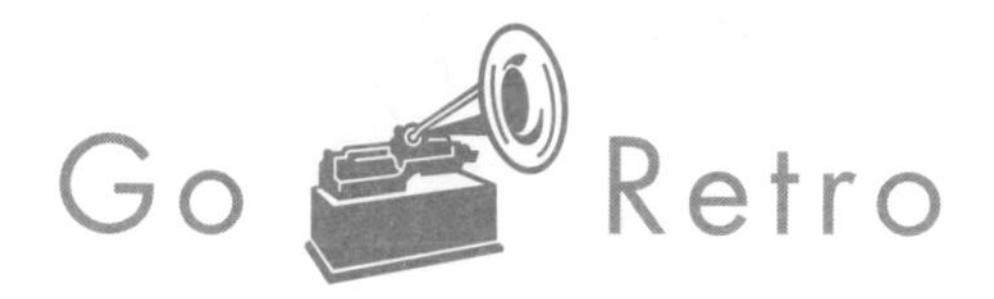

Get out those old 33 rpm records. A musical friend assures me that records have been scientifically proven to provide a more soothing sound to the ear than CDs and cassettes. Remember Johnny Mathis, Judy Collins, the Beatles? Turn on the record player and groove to your old favorites.

"Finish each day and be done with it. You have done what you could. Tomorrow is a new day; begin it well and serenely and with too high a spirit to be encumbered with your old nonsense."

Ralph Waldo Emerson

Practice the Cat Stretch

This wonderful yoga stretch, which increases flexibility and improves breathing, gets its inspiration from the sensual, expansive curls of a cat.

1. Get down on all fours with your hands directly under your shoulders and your knees right under your hips (the "table position").
2. Breathe out, slowly rounding your back up and gently dropping your chin to your chest. Continue to breathe and hold the position for a count of 5.
3. Breathe in, raising your head and slowly uncurling so that your back is slightly arched and you are looking straight ahead. Hold for a count of 5.
4. Repeat 5 times. Purr-fect!

Carry an Umbrella

Being prepared minimizes stress. So purchase a few small, fold-up umbrellas. Leave one in your car, another in your attaché or at the office. Then you'll never worry about getting caught in the rain.

Are you constantly looking at your watch while **WAITING** in line at the supermarket? Are you impatient before an appointment or until your children's lessons are finished? Treat yourself to a "waiting enhancer." Carry a favorite magazine or paper-back book in your bag to while away the time pleasantly.

Take a jog or an **AEROBICS** class. More than 70 percent of people say that they don't work out because they are too tired, but what they may not know is that exercise is a great stress reliever. If you break the fatigue–inactivity cycle, you will be rewarded with relaxation.

Bath and Shower Combo

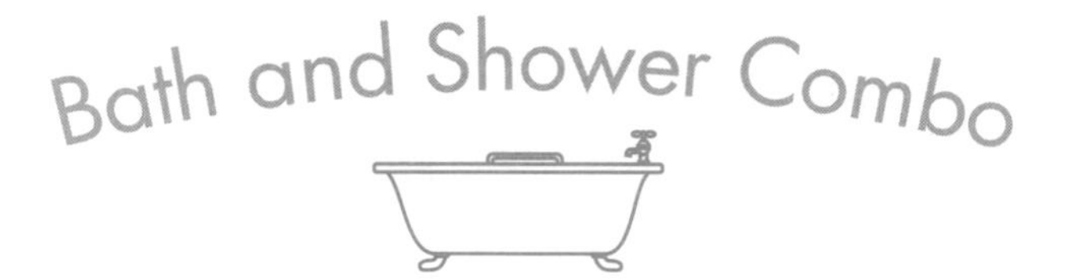

After a tiring day, soothe those tight muscles by filling the bathtub with 2 cups of Epsom salts and hot water (stimulating, but not scalding). Sink into the tub and lounge with a towel or bath pillow behind your head. When the water begins to cool, stand up and turn on the shower. Rinse off with a blast of cold water, then end with a warming stream.

AROMA THERAPY

Essential oils are highly concentrated essences derived from plants and flowers. Relax with the sedating scents of lavender, lemon balm, Roman chamomile, neroli, ylang ylang, and clary sage.

Postpone Procrastination

We often put off unpleasant tasks. We stall because we are afraid of making decisions or mistakes. This just prolongs our tension and discomfort. Figure out the reasons for your procrastination. Then, don't delay. Do it now!

Write your own **HOROSCOPE.** Some mornings don't you just wish the overgeneralized newspaper horoscopes were right? Make believe. "Grab the brass ring and do what you have wanted to do for a long time," or "The stars are right for romance." Live today with that possibility.

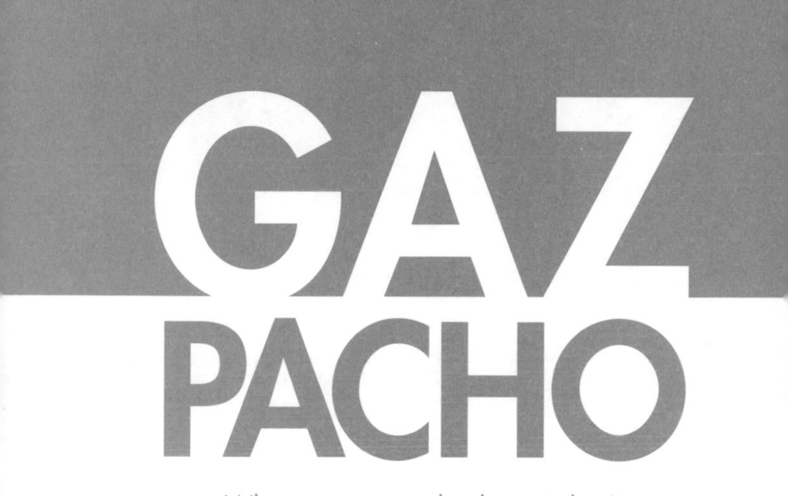

Who wants to cook when it's hot? Partnered with bakery-bought bread, cold soups are simple and satisfying summer fare. Try chilled gazpacho, a spicy Spanish vegetable soup prepared in a blender.

Schedule Worry

Schedule a worry session. If you honor your concerns for a focused half-hour, you may eliminate being plagued by worries throughout the day. Reserve a quiet time and place to sit and worry. Then, when you feel distressed outside of the specified time, say to yourself, "Don't worry now. I have plenty of time to worry later."

What does relaxation mean to you? How do you feel when you are relaxed? Write a list of relaxing words on an index card and keep it at your desk as a reminder. Here are some to start you off — calm, **PEACEFUL,** quiet, blissful, still, comfortable, mellow, tranquil, warm, slow, easy, refreshed.

"If you take your time and keep your wits about you, you can cultivate a wholesome and artful spiritual life that nourishes the whole self — one that will help you enjoy the world and perhaps even save it."

Elizabeth Lesser

Give Yourself a Hand

. . . a hand massage, that is. Using the thumb and index finger of your left hand, squeeze each finger on your right hand, one by one. Make rolling movements from your knuckles to your fingertips. Gently pull each finger, then switch hands.

Play Some Peaceful "Mind Movies"

Visualization engages your calm, creative center. Imagine a peaceful lake. Paint a picture with all of your senses. See the water's shimmering ripples, feel the gentle breeze, hear the call of the loons, and smell the fresh air. Picture yourself sitting there alone, breathing slowly and enjoying the tranquillity of the outdoors. Take this sense of serenity with you as you continue with your day.

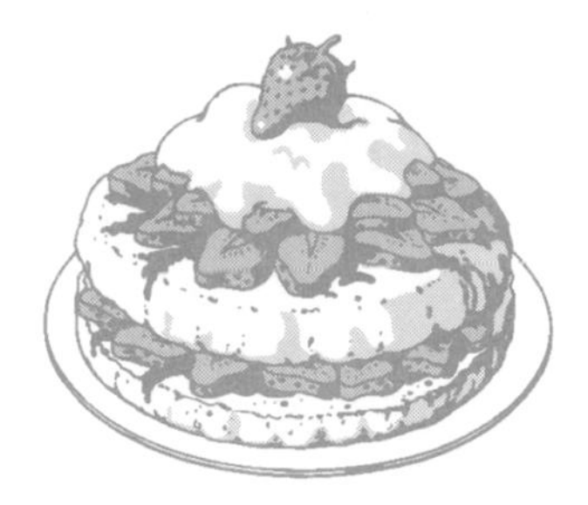

Eat dessert first.
The strawberries
are ripe and the
shortcake is made.
Why wait?

Plan a Celebration

Imagine a silly but special celebration. If you're the dramatic type, celebrate the Academy Awards, either by yourself or with a couple of close friends. Don your fanciest clothes and serve an elegantly simple spread. Smoked oysters, anyone? If you love Goofy and the rest of the Disney gang, make sure that they are represented at your birthday celebrations. What will you wear and what specialties will you serve?

Let the morning sun **SHINE** on you. Bright natural light early in the day enhances your body's internal rhythms and helps you sleep better at night.

Sing Your Own Song

What song best reflects your personal goals? What piece of music could help you maintain your calm center during a hectic day? Try humming your favorite tune before a dreaded meeting or sing your chosen song in the shower or car. Who knows? Soon you may hear those around you tapping to your beat.

Enjoy a Magical Drink

To many New Yorkers, egg creams are more than drinks — they evoke the wonder of childhood, and sipping one brings back memories of slower days. Actually, egg creams don't contain any eggs or cream and are only a fancy fizzed version of chocolate milk!

MAKES 1 SERVING

- 3 tablespoons chocolate syrup
- ⅓ cup ice-cold milk
- ⅔ cup seltzer

1. Pour the chocolate syrup into a tall glass.
2. Add the milk and stir.
3. Fill the rest of the glass with the seltzer while stirring. You've got it right when the top third of the glass is thickly foamed.

Shed Your Scarlet Letter

Letting go of an old regret or shameful memory is often difficult but always liberating. What would help you heal? How can you shed the weight of a past transgression? Write about it in your journal. Or find a truly sympathetic person to share your secret with — a friend, support-group member, or counselor.

VALERIAN is the premier herb to treat insomnia and stress. German studies have proven its benefits as a relaxant without sedative side effects. When valerian is paired with the more pleasant-tasting lemon balm, its strong odor is masked while its relaxing qualities are enhanced. Try this combination in liquid extracts or capsules.

Child's Pose

This gentle reclining yoga position is relaxing and will help you sleep better.

1. Kneel on the floor. Spread your knees shoulder-width apart while keeping your feet together. Lower your buttocks onto your heels.
2. Bend forward. Lower your chest to your knees.
3. Place your head on the floor with your face turned to one side or with your forehead resting on the ground.
4. Rest for a few minutes with your arms by your sides and your palms up. Breathe slowly and deeply.

Food of the Gods

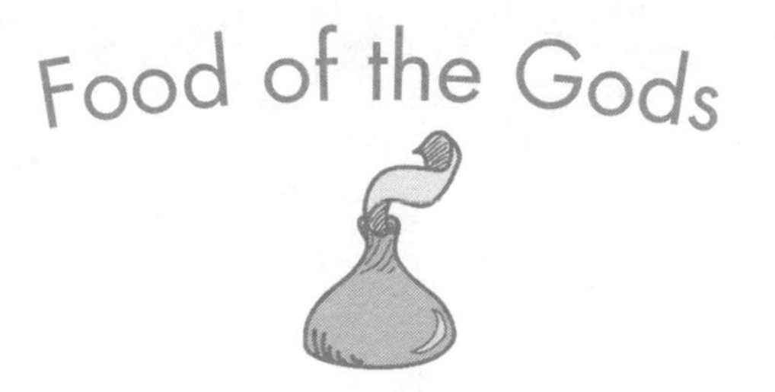

Recent studies suggest that there is no reason to feel guilty about your craving for chocolate. A dietary source of magnesium, chocolate contains antioxidants and heart-healthy compounds. Even if it weren't so good for you, a delicious chocolate treat is relaxing.

Enjoy a Trashy Novel

Don't be embarrassed — reading sappy, silly, or simple books is a wonderful form of no-stress entertainment. So cruise over to the library or bookstore and stock up! Books with "no redeeming value" are golden for lying on the couch on a cold winter's day or for packing in your beach bag for a summer idyll.

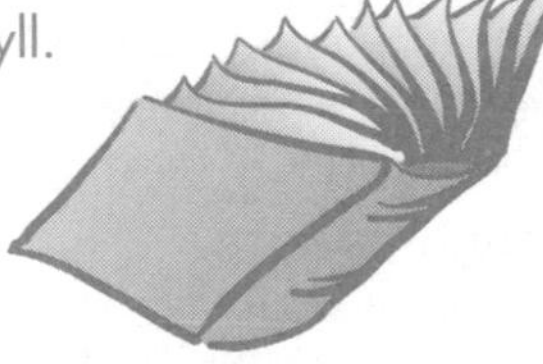

RE
MEMBER

Relive pleasant memories.
Save some favorite cards and letters
to reread while sipping a cup of tea.
Appreciate the connections and comfort
of your larger community.

"Moving toward an inwardly simple life is not about deprivation or denying ourselves the things we want. It's about getting rid of the things that no longer contribute to the fullness of our lives. It's about creating balance between our inner and outer lives."

Elaine St. James

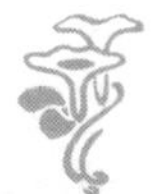

Lavender Lullaby

It's easy and relaxing to make and use bath salts at home.

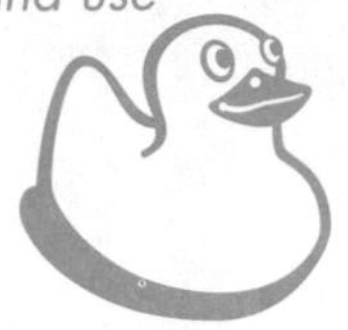

⅓ cup baking soda
⅓ cup Epsom salts
⅓ cup sea salt
10 drops lavender essential oil

1. In a nonporous bowl, combine the baking soda, Epsom salts, and sea salt. Add the lavender essential oil.
2. Cover the mixture with a cotton cloth and leave it to dry overnight.
3. In the morning, stir the mixture to break up any chunks. Store it in a pretty bottle or tin.

To use, pour ½ cup of the salts into the tub as it is filling with warm water.

Relaxation is contagious. Spend time with calm companions.

Lessen your holiday stress by **LIMITING** gifts to a pre-planned amount. Enhance the spiritual meaning of the season while eliminating credit card debt.

Connect with Nature

At the first sign of spring, take a hike in the woods or a walk on the beach. Seasonal relaxation engages the senses. Where can you go to renew your connection with the healing power of the earth?

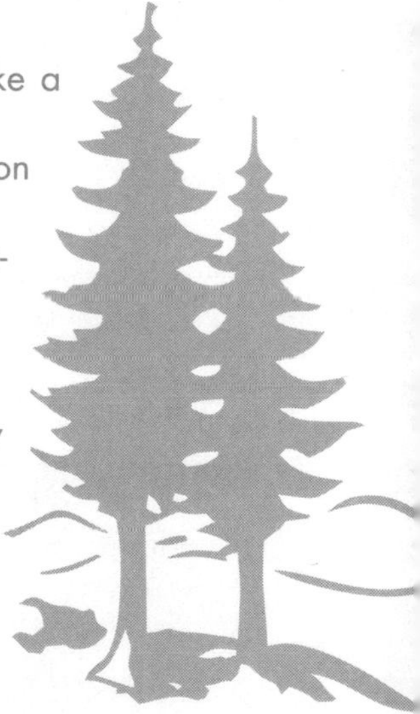

Develop a New Way of Seeing

A creative teacher used this technique to help his students gain a new visual perspective. Add one drop of red ink to a full glass of water and you might see an angel, rubies, or a favorite relative. Stop, look around you, and change one small detail. The new things you observe may surprise you.

Turn Off the Television

The majority of American families spend more time watching TV every day than they do speaking to each other. If you're not ready to eliminate all TV time, try to cut your viewing by half. Fill the extra time chatting with family members or just enjoying the newfound silence.

MONO POLY

Before video games and computers,
folks relaxed together around the game board.
Dust off those old favorites hiding in the back
of the cabinet or purchase new ones
for some Friday evening fun.

Choose a **COMFORTING** commuting companion. Garrison Keillor produces the Writer's Almanac, a quirky five-minute morning show on National Public Radio. Are country songs more to your liking? How about a local talk-show personality who makes you laugh? Invite someone along on your morning drive.

Go Fly a Kite

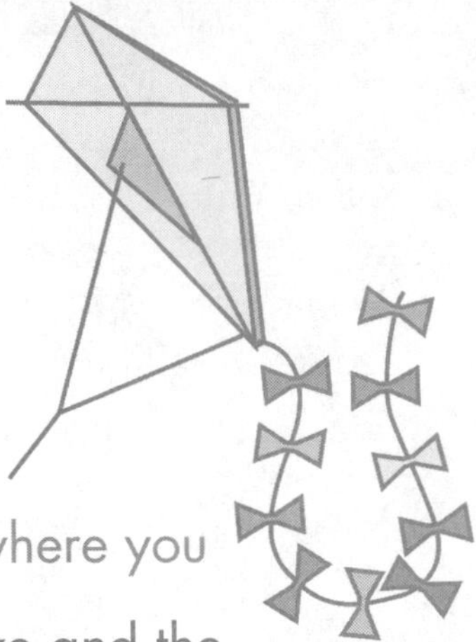

Find relaxing fun in a windy field where you can feel the breeze and the freedom of flight.

Centering Breath

Feeling anxious and out-of-sorts? Come back to yourself with this breathing exercise.

1. Place the index and middle fingers of your left hand horizontally across your chin and press gently.
2. At the same time, place the index and middle fingers of your right hand 2 inches below your navel and press.
3. Drop your shoulders and take four deep breaths. (This can also help stop a case of the hiccups.)

Don't be a victim of your hairdo! Consult with a talented hairstylist and choose a **VERSATILE** wash-and-wear style that looks attractive and lessens morning primp time. Bring magazine pictures to the salon to showcase the right look.

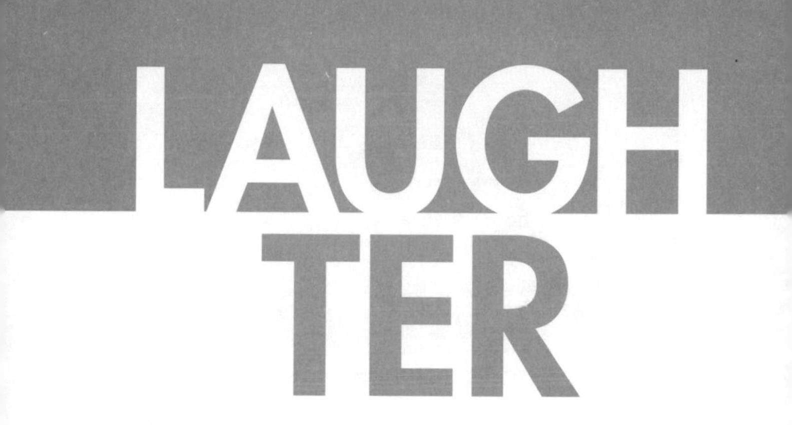

Humor is healing, and a night of laughter is good for the soul. Watch *I Love Lucy* reruns and videotapes of original funny favorites, such as Laurel and Hardy or Charlie Chaplin.

Reduce Road Rage

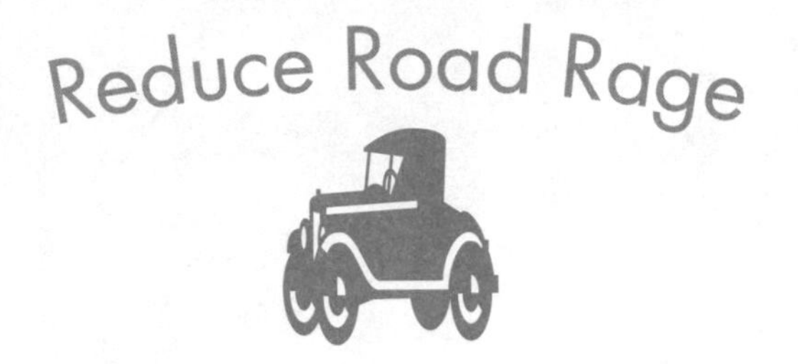

Anticipate traffic jams and the driving habits of other people. When possible, adjust your travel time to eliminate rush hour. Don't distract yourself by talking on a cellular phone; instead, calm down by listening to Sylvia Boorstein's *Road Sage* on audio cassette.

Live with a **POEM** for a week. Recite it daily. Reflect on the questions and meanings your chosen poem inspires. Poet Mary Oliver provides interesting food for thought when she asks, "What is it you plan to do with your one wild and precious life?"

Shoulder Shrugs

Don't carry the weight of the world; shrug it off! Shoulder shrugs are easy stretches that release tension from your upper body. You can do them while either sitting or standing.

1. Inhale and tighten your shoulders, pulling them up toward your ears.
2. Exhale and gently release.
3. Repeat three times.

Flower Essences

Rescue Remedy, a flower essence developed by Dr. Edward Bach in the 1930s, is a calming and stabilizing treatment for stress and trauma. This five-flower formula is nontoxic, nonaddictive, and free from any known side effects. Take it in small doses throughout a stressful day. Rescue Remedy is available at health food stores and natural pharmacies.

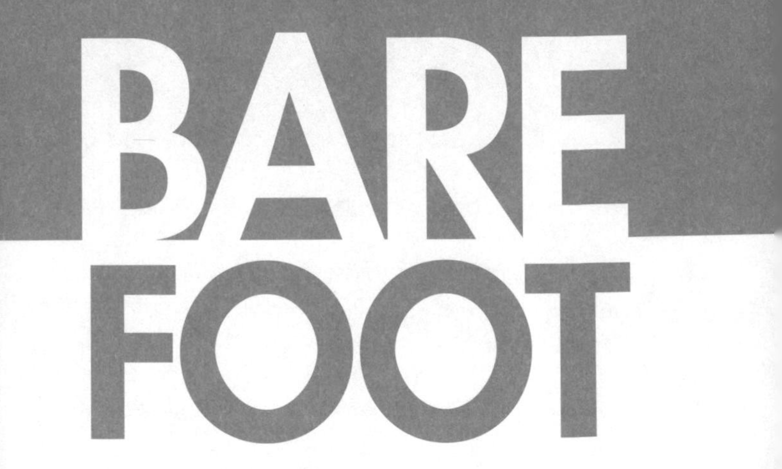

You don't have to tiptoe through the tulips to appreciate the many different textures under your feet. Indoor rugs and outdoor grass can soothe your sole.

"You must learn to be still in the midst of activity and to be vibrantly alive in repose."

Indira Gandhi

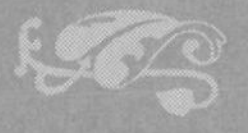

Plan a personal **PAMPERING** party. Turn off the phone, sift through a pile of magazines, give yourself a manicure, write a letter, loll in the bath, and plan your next creative endeavor.

Swan Stretch

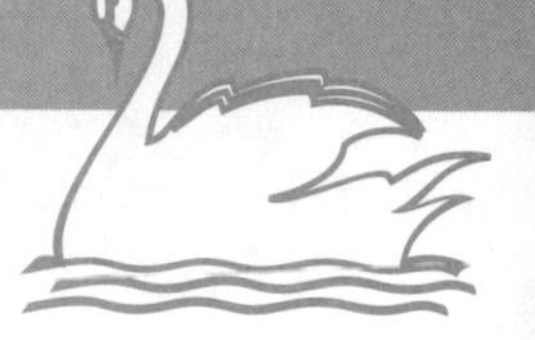

This stretch helps release chronic tension and gracefully lengthens your neck.

1. Sit in a cross-legged position on the floor with your back straight and your hands resting on your thighs.
2. Stretch your right arm out to the side and touch the floor with your right hand.
3. Inhale and stretch your head to the left. Don't lean forward. Feel the stretch from your head to your hands.
4. Exhale and release any tension into the ground through your fingers.
5. Inhale and straighten your head while returning your right hand to your thigh.
6. Repeat on the other side.

Slow Down with Soup

Start lunch with a bowl of soup. Soup sipping encourages slower meals. Studies show that people who begin their meals with soup consume fewer calories.

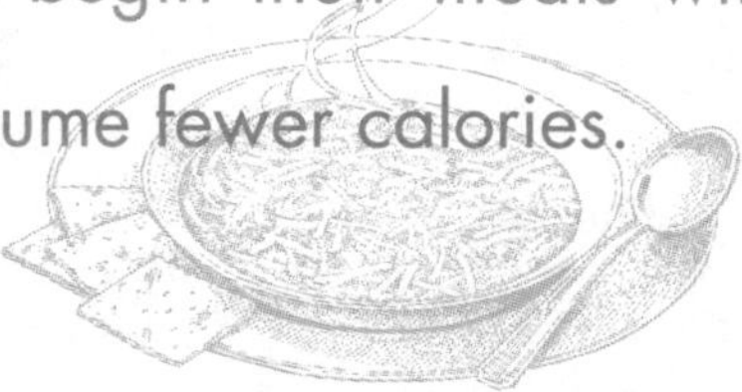

Describe the most **PLEASANT** and relaxing time you've ever experienced. Were you at home, on vacation, at a spa, or on a retreat? Were you alone or with others? What were you wearing and what did you eat? Do one small thing today that reminds you of that peaceful time.

Relaxing Massage Oil

It's easy to make your own massage oil for treating tense muscles.

4 teaspoons sweet almond oil
5 drops lavender essential oil
5 drops sandalwood essential oil

1. Combine the ingredients.
2. Apply the oil blend to tense muscles with long flowing strokes.

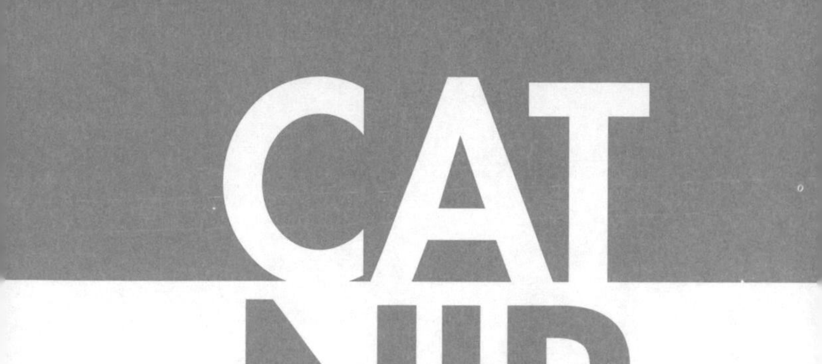

CAT NIP

Be an herbal copycat with catnip.
Catnip-stuffed toys may stimulate your feline,
but the herb has the opposite effect on people.
Catnip, a tasty and easy-to-grow
cousin of mint, makes a mild sedative tea.

Designate today as your personal **AROMA** day. Switch gears by stretching your sense of smell. Ask yourself these three questions: Which scents delight me? Which aromas relax me? What might I smell today?

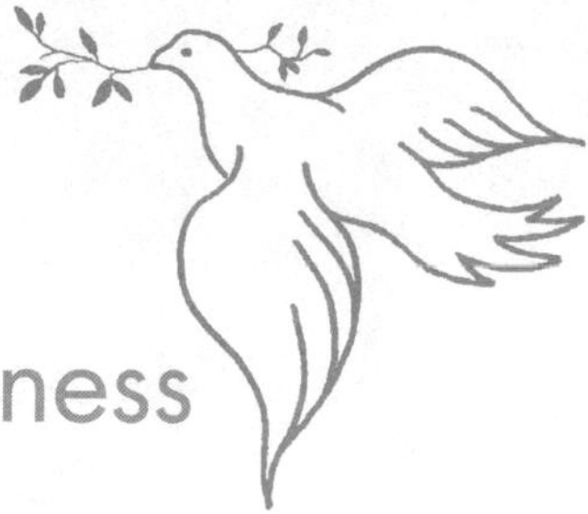

Cultivate a Heart of Stillness

Find a deep sense of inner peace by recommitting to your house of worship or finding a new spiritual home through a church group or personal prayer.

“A rich
world of wonder
awaits.”

Carl Sagan

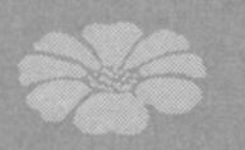

MEDITATION

Seek the secrets of silence.
Meditation teaches us how to quiet our overactive brains and experience a sense of serenity. Books, tapes, and classes can help you learn this potent method of self-observation.

Chew Slowly

Be conscious of each portion of food you put in your mouth and put your fork down in between bites.

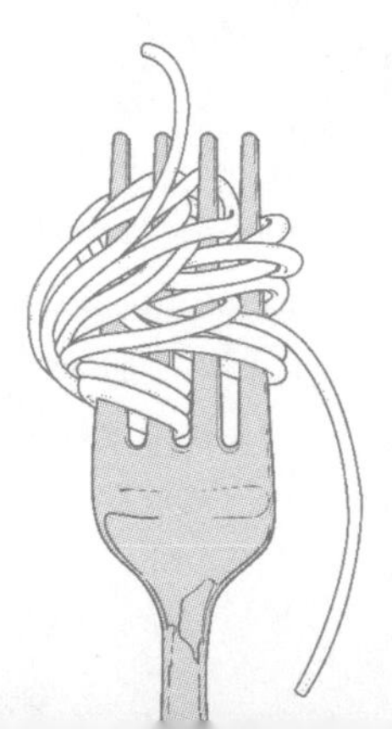

Pop singer Paul Simon once crooned, "Everyone loves the sound of a train in the distance." Listen to the **RHYTHMIC** clacking of a train and the whistle marking its approach. You can't hurry the train. Just notice it and breathe slowly until its music fades away.

Give Yourself a Time Cushion

Dreaded deadlines increase stress. For any pending project, pencil in your planner a personal deadline that is days or weeks before the actual deadline. If the computer crashes or you get a cold, you'll have the relief of extra time.

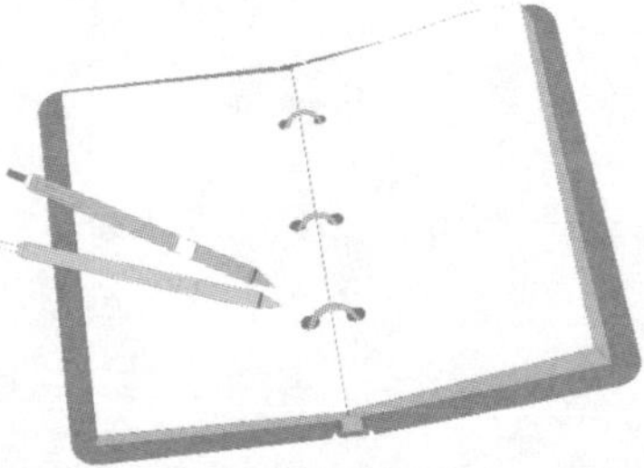

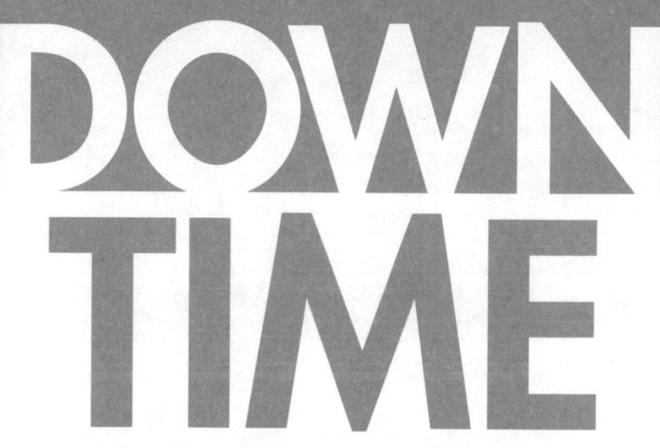

Pace yourself for a peaceful day.
Be aware of the time of day when you are most alert. Schedule that time to tackle creative or difficult tasks. Allot languid times for easier activities.

Simmer a small amount of cloves, **CINNAMON,** and orange peel, in two cups of water on top of the stove. The soothing fragrance will fill your home.

Nose Alphabets

Here's a quick way to ease tense neck muscles.

1. Sit up straight with your head forward and your shoulders relaxed.
2. Move your nose in small, smooth movements to trace the alphabet in the air — half-inch capital letters are best.

You may get some strange looks, but when others find out about this simple relaxing exercise, they may join you.

Don't Hold Your Breath

When "breathless" in anticipation or "frozen with fear," your breathing becomes shallow. Alleviate your anxiety by consciously altering the rhythm and depth of your breathing. Put one hand on your chest and the other on your abdomen. Create a quiet wave between your chest and belly by slowing and deepening your breath.

"Beauty of style
and harmony
and grace
and good rhythm
depend on
simplicity."

Plato

Travel Light

Lugging heavy and bulky luggage is stressful. Instead, choose a few mix-and-match outfits and pack a small rolling valise and a matching carry-on bag.

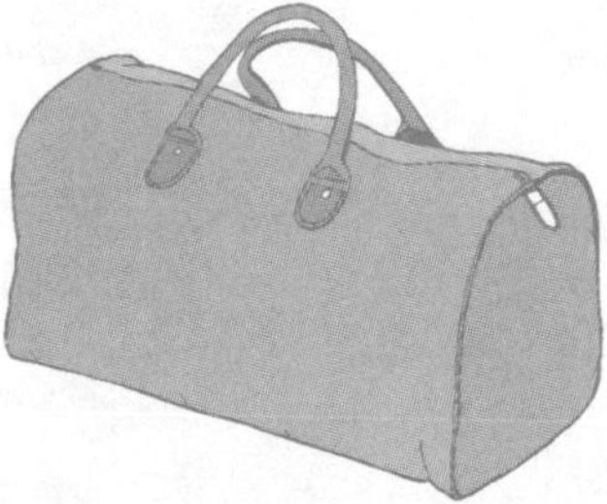

CHOREOGRAPHY

Lose those shoes and loosen your tie.
Choreograph your own calm
by moving to a slow tempo. Five minutes
on your feet followed by five minutes of
sitting still is a great stress reducer.

Don't Stifle That Sigh

As renowned yoga instructor Lillias Folan observed, "We have too many unsighed sighs inside of us." Let yours out. An audible exhalation acknowledges and releases tension.

Ahhhh

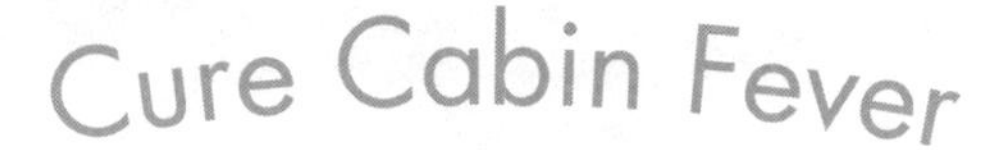

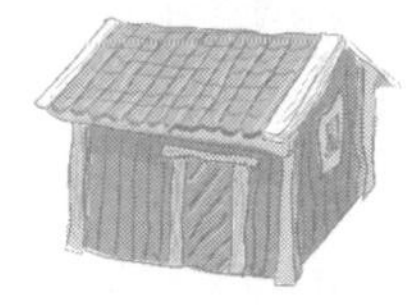

Coffee-table books cure cabin fever. They can transport you to the tropics during the winter or take you someplace cool and breezy when it's hot and humid outside. Try oversized library books full of photos for inspiration. Or browse through *National Geographic* and travel magazines.

The Lion Pose

Roars are relaxing. Let one out while practicing the Lion Pose, a tension-relieving yoga position.

1. Sit quietly with your eyes closed. Inhale through your nose.
2. Open your mouth wide and stick out your tongue. Stretch it down toward your chin.
3. Stretch your eyes into a wide stare; look up.
4. Let out a roar as you loudly exhale.
5. Close your mouth and relax your eyes. Repeat.

Cure Keyboard Cramps

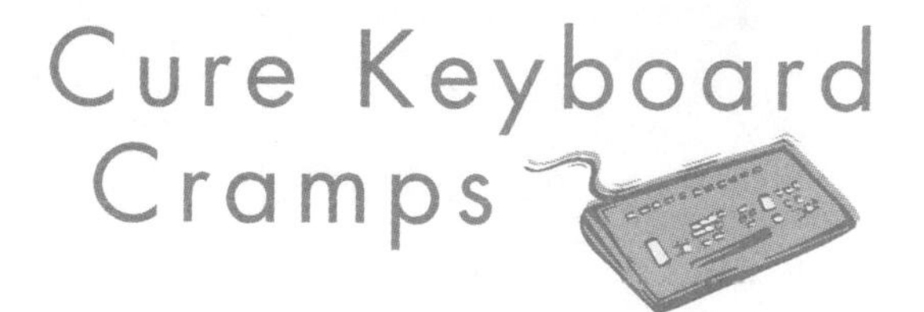

Sitting at the computer for hours encourages slouching and muscle cramps. To release tension, take short breaks and change your position hourly. Push your chair back and close your eyes or stand up and stretch.

Lighten Your Load

Cleaning out your closets lessens the amount you have to organize, clean, and repair. And that frees up time to relax.

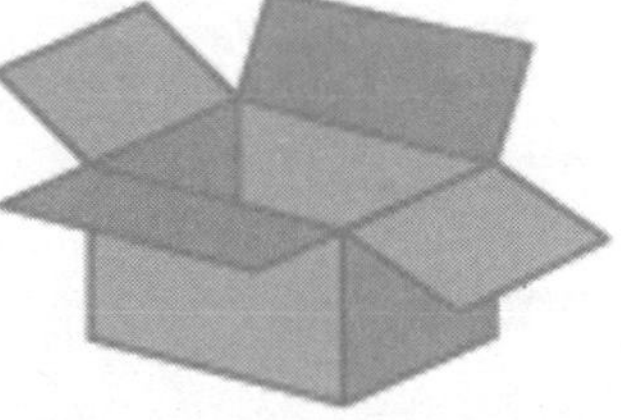

Forget "No pain, no gain." Instead, try **SMOOTH** stretching movements. Resist the tendency to bounce or push past discomfort. Breathe deeply while gently loosening. Repeat similar movements on both sides of your body.

RELAX ATION

How many words
can you make with the letters
from the word relaxation?

Don't Bring Work Home

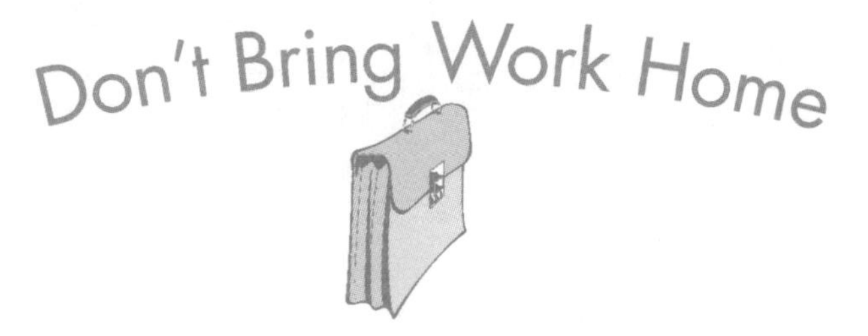

Make a transition at your front door. Purge the cares of the day by paring down overly practical and technological details. Don't allow your bedroom to do double duty as a mini-office. Put your desk and computer in another room or screen them from view with a pretty room divider.

Find Relaxation Role Models

Who seems to live the calm, balanced life that you crave? Ask the people you admire how they do it. You may be surprised by their challenges and helped by their resources, tools, and ideas.

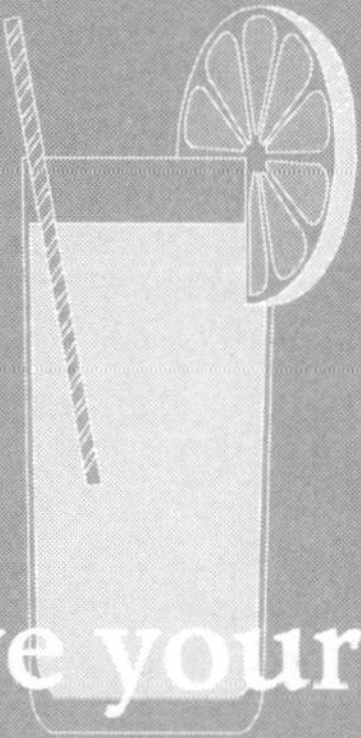

Serve yourself
a glass of
ice-cold lemonade
and sip it
through a straw.

Find an antidote for the "Arsenic Hour," the stressful period before dinner. Tame this tense time with an array of preplanned activities and guidelines for the kids. Have on hand some **SIMPLE** nutritious snacks, such as carrot sticks or cheese and crackers. Limit telephone and television use and play some **QUIET** background music instead.

Brush Your Hair

Tradition recommends 100 strokes nightly, but gently brushing your hair without counting may be more relaxing. To encourage healthy hair growth and enhance thickness, add 1 or 2 drops of rosemary essential oil to your hairbrush.

POP CORN

Invite your family or friends
to a movie marathon — at home.
Combine some classics with new releases.
Pass the popcorn.

Keep your hands busy and the rest of you will **SLOW DOWN.** Devote 15 minutes daily to needlework. Stitch a serene scene preprinted on canvas. Starter kits are available at craft stores. To prolong the relaxation benefits, display the finished piece in your work area.

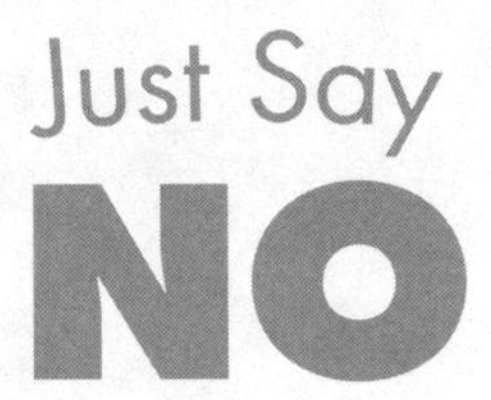

Overloaded with too many tasks, we still often agree to one more responsibility. This month pass on all requests for your participation. Clearing the decks will help you decide what is most important to you. And remember, next month when you are calm and centered, you can agree to serve on that committee.

Hold That Pose

Stop and become aware of your posture. Are you slumped in your chair? Feeling tense or tight? If so, don't quickly change positions. Exhale fully and gently exaggerate your stance. Then inhale and slowly straighten.

Self-Massage

Prolonged desk work causes tight shoulders and upper arms. Take a minibreak and rub the stress away with a self-massage.

1. Place your left hand on your right shoulder.
2. Gently knead the muscles between your neck and arm.
3. Squeeze. Hold for a few seconds, then release.
4. Continue to gently squeeze and rub along your shoulder and upper arm.
5. Repeat on your left side.

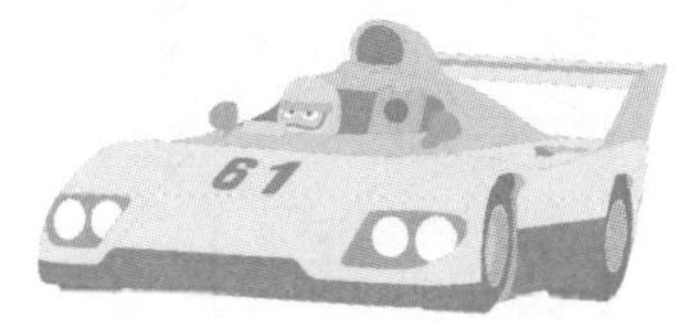

Curb Competitive Commuting

White knuckles on the wheel and a lead foot on the pedal may get you there a bit faster — but you'll also be frazzled. Getting to work shouldn't be a race. Allow 5 to 10 extra minutes for your morning drive.

Listen for the sounds of the seasons. Autumn is marked by honking geese announcing their departure for warmer climes; the red robin's morning song signals spring. Wherever you live, whether city, suburb, or countryside, notice how nature's music changes throughout the year.

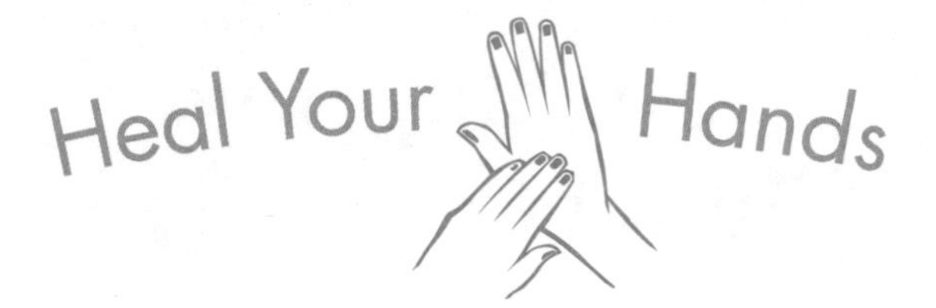

Heal Your Hands

When your hands are overused and underappreciated, they're at risk for strain injuries. Be sure to take breaks from typing and other tasks that require repetitive hand movements. Wiggle your fingers, then stretch them wide apart. Make a fist with your whole hand and release it. Then gently shake the tension out of your hands.

As the song goes, "Summertime and the living is easy." That's when meal preparation should be quick and **UNCOMPLICATED.** Have a salad for supper on a summer's eve. Eat on the porch or picnic in the park.

Turn Off the Alarm Clock

If you need an alarm to wake up, you are probably sleep deprived. This week-end, catch up on needed rest and wake up naturally.

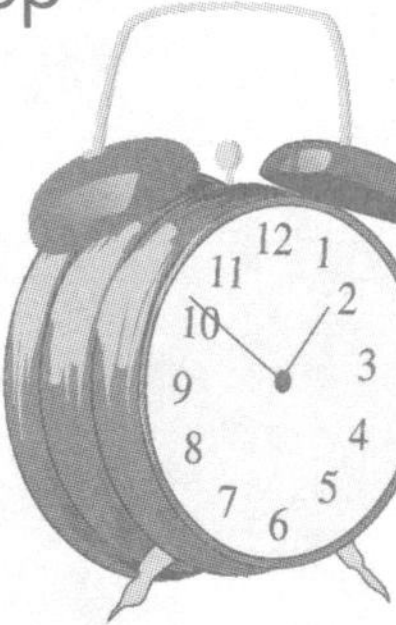

Headache Tamer

Tame tension headaches with this simple massage technique.

1. Place your index and middle fingers of both hands at the outer edges of your eyebrows and on the indentations at your temples.

2. Rub in small circular movements.

3. Increase the pressure and hold for a count of 2.

4. Release; repeat as necessary.

"There will
be time enough
to do it all.
But not all at once."

Wayne Sotile

Toss Out Time Wasters

When we're tired and tense, we often choose time-wasting activities that don't rejuvenate us. Replace Web surfing with listening to a tape of soothing music or doing a half-hour of yoga. Free up your free time for some really relaxing activities.

Heads Down

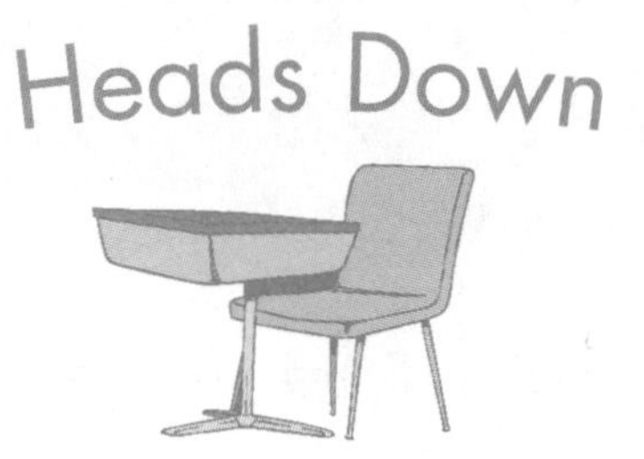

Elementary school teachers have the right idea when they tell their classes how best to relax. It works for adults, too! Push your chair back. Lean forward from your waist. Rest your forehead on your folded arms on your desk. Your productivity and creativity will get a jump start with a five-minute break.

Share the work and savor the **LEISURE** time. Make sure that everyone on your home team is responsible for his or her own area. Even young children can do simple chores. Older family members can do their own laundry, and dinner preparation can be rotated.

"Be willing to live in between right and wrong. The ego needs and desperately wants to be right and make others wrong. In between right and wrong is a soft, messy, laughing place where it doesn't matter."

SARK

Seashell Meditation

Save some seashells from the beach. Bring them home and relive the serenity of the seashore with this simple meditation.

1. Place a seashell in front of you. Sit quietly and pay attention to your breathing.
2. Gaze at the shell. Move your eyes around its curves.
3. Sense the shell without describing it. When words or judgments pop up, just let them pass.
4. Sit like this for 5 to 10 minutes before you return to other activities.

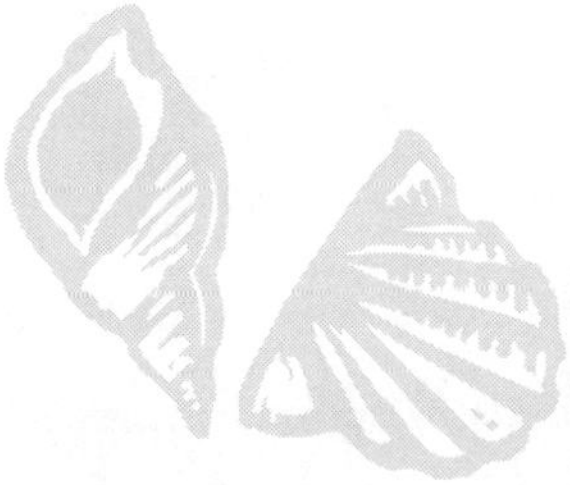

Designate today as your personal **SIGHT** day. Release your thoughts and worries by stretching your sense of sight. Ask yourself these three questions: Which sights delight me? Which sights relax me? What might I see today?

Value Evocative Vanilla

Vanilla's deep, sweet scent summons a sense of calm. Light a vanilla-scented candle, moisturize with a vanilla lotion, or add a dash of pure vanilla extract to your cup of decaffeinated coffee.

Play with Clay

Get your hands dirty; pottery making is an acceptable way to make a mess. Squeezing and molding clay releases tension. You can make functional or abstract pieces right at your kitchen table with a variety of products that you can bake or dry naturally. Or sign up for a beginner's pottery class.

Simplify holiday gift giving. Instead of searching for the perfect gift, choose a **THEME,** such as books or kitchen supplies, and buy similar presents for everyone on your list.

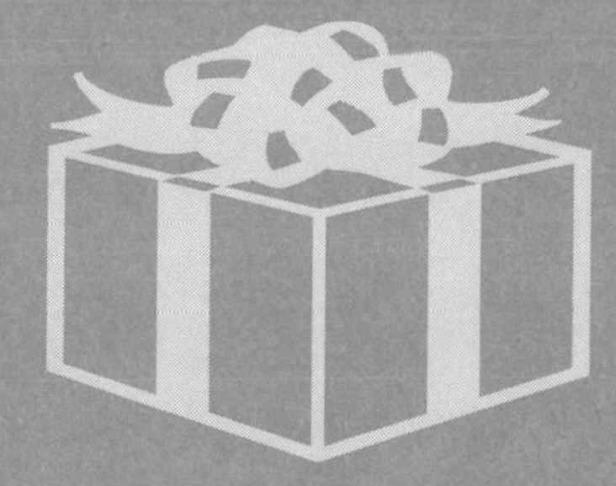

Get out of your chair and do the **TWIST.** Stand face forward with your feet comfortably apart. Bend your knees slightly. Swing your arms backward and forward across your body several times. With or without music, this **TEMPO** will help you release tension.

Create Calm with Crystals

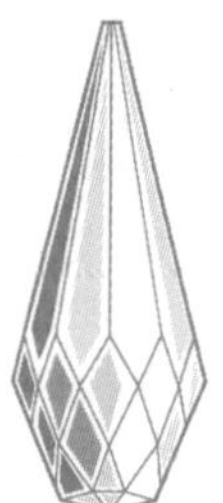

Crystals are beautiful and have various healing potentials. Amethyst is calming and soothing; quartz is balancing. Display the crystals in your bedroom, family room, or meditation area.

Don't Cheat Sleep

The average adult needs seven to nine hours of sleep a night to function well. Most Americans get only six hours of sleep or less. Insufficient sleep is both physically and psychologically stressful. An extra 45 minutes of sleep can increase your immunity and improve your overall well-being.

KAVA KAVA is an ancient ceremonial and medicinal herb from the South Pacific islands. It's a wonderful remedy for mild to moderate anxiety. Health food stores and natural pharmacies stock capsules and extracts. Follow label directions.

"If trying harder
doesn't work,
try softer."

Lily Tomlin

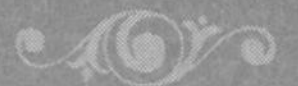

Take a Slow Shower

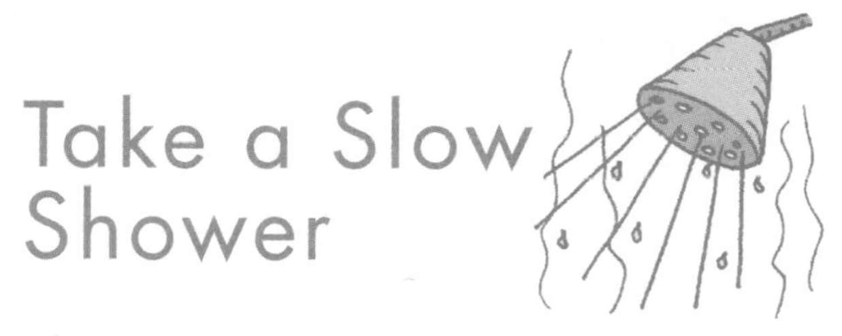

Showers are mistakenly viewed as the stimulating sibling of the sedative bath. But steamy showers can be sensual and relaxing. Linger and let the water massage your tense muscles.

Select Comfortable Bedding

After a tiring day, ensure yourself a foundation of rest. Indulge in comfortable bedding, such as a downy comforter and a large mattress. Sink into the caresses of a feather bed. Buy the softest sheets you can afford. Choose cool, all-cotton sheets in the summer and try a set of flannel sheets to keep you warm on winter nights. Sleep in your own cradle of comfort.

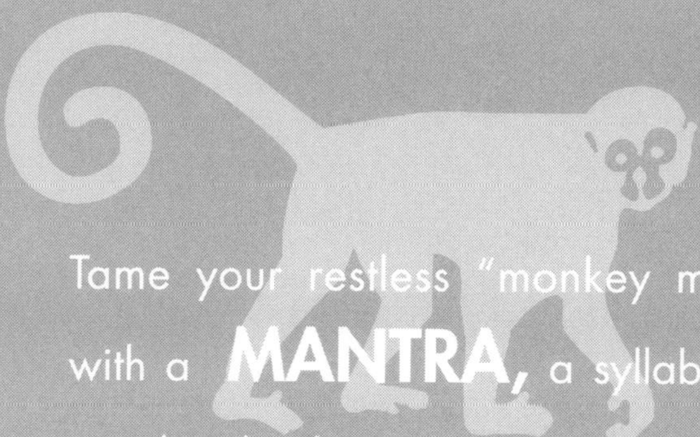

Tame your restless "monkey mind" with a **MANTRA,** a syllable or word silently repeated or softly spoken during meditation. Intoning "peace," "relax," "om," or "one" will slow down your overactive mind.

Take a Walk

A sleep survey found that those who walked at least six blocks a day at a normal pace were one-third less likely to have trouble sleeping than nonwalkers. Those who walked faster decreased their risk of sleep disorders by 50 percent. If you are enlisting exercise as a sleep aid, afternoon workouts have the most benefit; don't exercise within three to five hours of bedtime.

Sleepy Time Bath Bags

Try this recipe for a soothing, sleep-inducing bath.

MAKES 6 BATH BAGS

1 cup dried chamomile flowers
1 cup dried lavender flowers
½ cup dried hops
½ cup dried rose petals

1. Combine the ingredients.
2. Pour ½ cup of the mixture into small cotton or muslin drawstring bags.

When running the bath, loop the drawstring over the faucet so the water runs through the bag as the tub fills.

Acupressure Points

A handy way to relieve general aches and pains is to massage the pressure point on each palm.

1. Use the thumb and index finger of one hand to squeeze the soft tissue between the thumb and index finger of the other hand.
2. Press, hold for a count of 3, and release.
3. Repeat two times on each hand.

Avoid alcoholic beverages before **BEDTIME.** Although alcohol may help you doze off, its stimulant qualities disrupt deep sleep. Substitute an evening cup of warm milk or herbal tea for a hot toddy.

Have a Spa-rty

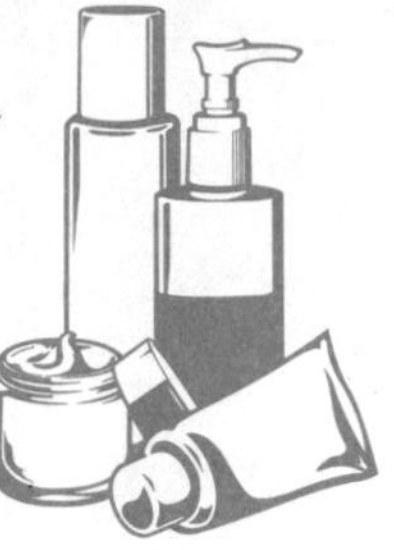

This is the adult version of a slumber party with a theme. Ask each guest to bring supplies for a spa treatment, such as hair conditioners, facials, and manicures. Share secrets while shampooing each other's hair.

Progressive Muscle Relaxation

Muscle relaxation and anxiety are incompatible. As you contract and release your muscles, you release stress.

1. Flex your left foot, then point your toes. Don't strain; continue to breathe slowly and deeply.
2. Hold for 5 seconds and then release. Repeat with your right foot.
3. Contract and release your calf, knee, and thigh muscles. Continue to tense, hold, and release. Alternate sides of your body.
4. Contract and release your groin and stomach area, your back, and your arms and hands.
5. Proceed to your neck, face, and head.
6. Rub your hands together and gently place your warm palms over your eyes.

Design a bedtime **RITUAL.** Reserve the last hour before bed for soaking in the bath, reading in a comfortable chair, and listening to instrumental music. This restful routine will help you release the day's concerns.

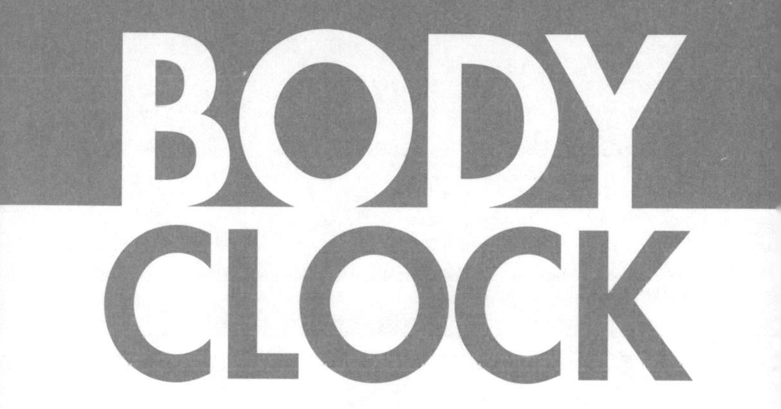

If you have problems sleeping,
reset your body clock by keeping to a curfew.
Go to bed at the same time every night
and get up at the same time every morning.

Spend time reading about a new-to-you field, such as science, historical fiction, relationships, or crafts. Choose a topic that you would like to learn more about, or find solace in a biography or fictional life story.

Eliminate Entertainment Pressure

Getting together with friends should be easy and enjoyable. Here are some guidelines for stress-free entertaining:

* Shop ahead and prepare ahead.
* Choose foods and dishes that require little cooking time.
* Don't try recipes for the first time.

Make a Sour Face

. . . it won't stay that way. Tightening and releasing facial muscles is relaxing and can keep tension headaches in check. Squeeze your eyes tight, scrunch your nose, and pucker your lips as if eating a sour lemon. Take a deep breath and release.

Create a Relaxation Haven

Keep a file of magazine pictures of serene bedrooms. Note the similarities in colors, shapes, and textures of rooms that appeal to you. Add some of these relaxing aspects to your own bedroom.

CARBO HYDRATES

Eat calming carbohydrates,
such as bread, cereal, and pasta,
to trigger the brain chemicals
that make you sleepy.

Select a Space for Quiet Time

Convert a cozy corner or empty room into a place to meditate. Choose a comfortable chair or cushion to sit on. Add a CD player for soft music or meditation tapes. Decorate the walls and floor with peaceful artwork. For privacy, separate the area from the rest of the house with gently flowing curtains or a screen.

"We embark upon the creation of a peaceful lifestyle by recognizing the need, daily, to cleanse our minds just as we cleanse our bodies. Through morning prayers and meditation, we embark upon the day spiritually prepared. Without this preparation, we enter the day with yesterday's anxieties — our own and those of millions of others."

Marianne Williamson

Transform your bedroom into a restful **SANCTUARY.** Reserve this room for sleeping, reflecting, and romancing. Surround yourself with dreamlike images. Eliminate flashy or distracting artwork, bedding, wall coverings, and window treatments. View only gentle beauty from your bed. This will enhance your mood and the quality of your sleep.

Visualization

This exercise can help you release your worries. Sit quietly and close your eyes. Picture a basket on your lap. Name your burdensome concerns, one by one, as you put them into the container. Imagine walking to a stream and pouring the basket's contents into the water. Watch your worries float away. And when you return to the real world, remember that the flowing water continues to carry your cares downstream.

Limit Violent Images

Popular action movies are rife with terror and mayhem. Eighty percent of all TV shows portray acts of aggression. This constant barrage of brutality stresses our minds and singes our souls. Instead, watch a comedy or nature show.

Desperately seeking **SERENITY** in all the wrong places? Ditch the Friday evening Happy Hour. Instead, take an end-of-the-week retreat. Plan ahead for some relaxing time alone. Order some healthy take-out food, pick up a good book or video, and get to bed early.

With no major investment, you can borrow a treasure from the vast book collection at your local library. Check out books about relaxation, meditation, and exercise.

Do One Thing at a Time

Time-management experts tell us that to get more done, we should "multitask." But this approach creates pressure and distraction. Instead, focus on one activity at a time. The next time you wash the dinner dishes, pay attention. Wash each one slowly and thoroughly. Completing one task at a time fosters inner serenity as well as true efficiency.

Ease the transition from work to home. Change into comfortable, casual clothes and leave your work concerns behind.

Mind Your Minerals

Make sure to get your share of calming calcium. In addition to building strong bones and teeth, calcium helps regulate healthy nerve and muscle function. A combination of calcium and magnesium acts as a mild relaxant and sleep promoter. Supplemental calcium also relieves premenstrual symptoms.

Don't rush. Remember, life is not a race. Allow yourself time to linger. Relaxation and satisfaction have space to grow only when we slow our pace.

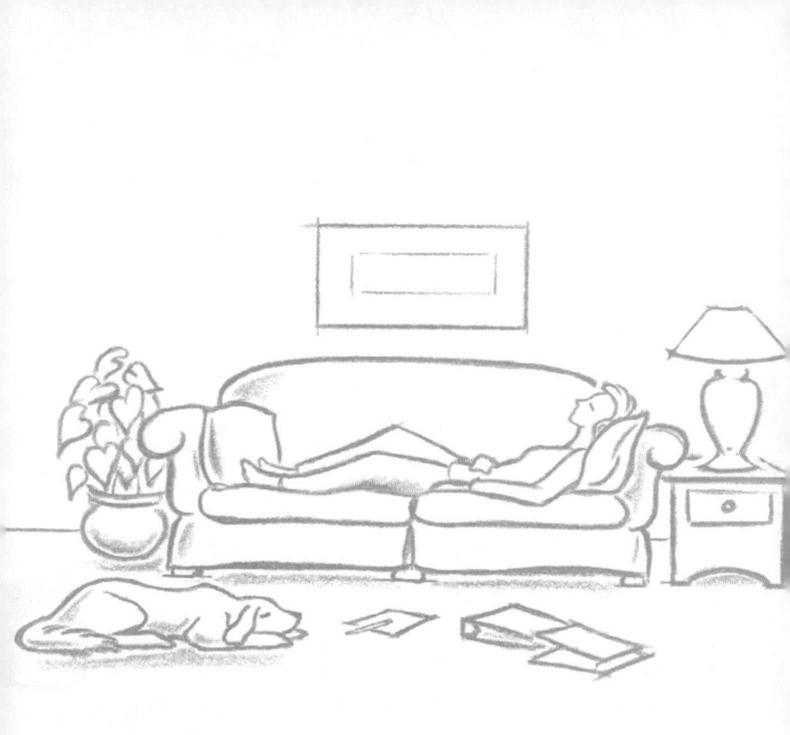

Take the Day Off

Remember your joy when school was closed due to bad weather? Don't wait for a storm or a bad cold to take a break. Reward yourself with a Mental Health Day. Cancel all your plans. And don't spend your time trying to catch up. Instead, luxuriate in winding down.

Cool as a Cucumber

Gently place slices of cool cucumber on your closed eyelids. Lie down for 5 minutes. This tension reliever has added visual effects — it temporarily reduces under-eye puffiness.

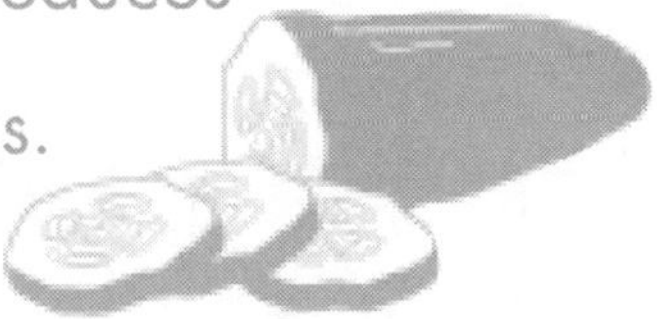

No Excuses

Sometimes we mutter the excuse, "If I could only get away, I could really relax." We jealously imagine how more fortunate people unwind in style. A famous actress, rich enough to travel to exotic places, revealed her favorite way to relax. She wakes late on a weekend morning and drinks a cup of specialty coffee while reading *The New York Times*. You, too, can create a simple, relaxing weekend ritual.

LAUGHTER

A good laugh is the "tranquilizer with no side effects." Laughing reduces stress hormone levels, decreases blood pressure, and relieves muscle tension. So yuk it up!

Don't Go Cold Turkey

You'll only get discouraged if you try to dump all your couch potato habits at once. Today, trade a half-hour of time-wasting TV for a walk. Or turn off the computer and turn on soft music instead.

Treat Your Feet

After being cooped up in shoes all day, these dogs need to dance.

1. Take off all foot coverings. Sit in a comfortable chair or lie down.
2. Alternately flex and extend each foot from the ankle.
3. Make five ankle circles with your right foot.
4. Change directions and do five more.
5. Repeat with your left foot.

Imagine an **IDEAL** morning. What time would you get out of bed? Who would be the first person to greet you? Would you make time to stretch or jog, write in your journal, or say morning prayers? Would you eat a light breakfast? Use your fantasies to design a **GRACEFUL** awakening.

Lounge in Lavender

This fragrant flower is a natural treatment for insomnia, nervousness, and headaches. Lather up with lavender soap or bath gel. If you have a headache, lie down with a lavender-scented compress. Add dried lavender to a cup of herbal tea or punch. And to ensure a restful evening, scent your sheets and pillow with a lavender spray.

Lazy Days

Appreciate the art of lazy days. Sleep late. Stroll to a bakery. Leisurely read the Sunday paper. Go window-shopping. You'll experience a tranquil transformation while you enjoy the most effortless activities.

On blustery winter nights, hunker down with a **HEARTY** stew. Lengthy meal preparation isn't relaxing. Instead, put a few simple ingredients in a pot and let them simmer away.

“There is
nothing
worth more
than this day.”

Johann Wolfgang von Goethe

Move Your Bed

According to the principles of feng shui, the ancient Oriental art of object placement, positioning your bed correctly can improve your sleep as well as your relationships. For optimum health, never put your bed in direct line with a door or a bathroom. Don't place your bed under beams and don't store items underneath your bed.

Socialize more while preparing less. Invite friends to an old-fashioned potluck. Ask everyone to bring a favorite dish to share. You supply the place, plates, flat-ware, beverages, and inviting atmosphere.

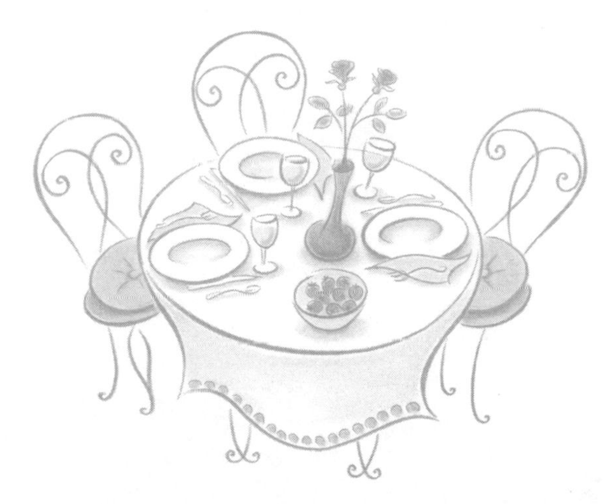

Squeeze Out Tension

Try this easy technique to relieve head and neck tension.

1. Place your left palm between your eyebrows and your right palm on the small indentation at the base of your skull.
2. Press and hold for a count of 5.
3. Release, relax for a moment, and then repeat two times.

Smudge Your Space

Smudging, or burning bundles of sweet-smelling herbs to cleanse odors and energy, is an ancient ritual. To clear the air, light a smudge stick made of sage or cedar. (A stick of incense is an acceptable substitute.) Hold the stick over a shell or a pretty bowl. Walk with it around the room. Waft the fragrant smoke from the floor to the ceiling, then relax in your sacred space.

If vacation travel is
not on the horizon,
treat yourself
to an afternoon in
"another world."
Take a solitary trip
to a café or bookstore
and leave the cellular
phone at home.

Communing with an animal is **RESTORATIVE.** The quality of life in nursing homes improves dramatically when pets come to play with the residents. Studies show that stroking a pet helps lower blood pressure. So curl up with a cat or dawdle with a dog.

Dehydration stresses the body. **Drink eight glasses of water every day** to help detoxify your blood and **eliminate wastes from your body.**

Go Fish

Gather your gear and head outdoors before the rest of the world wakes up. Stop focusing on all the other fish you have to fry and cast away your cares.

Sea Salt Body Scrub

Try this body scrub to soothe your senses and smooth your skin.

½ cup fine sea salt
¼ cup canola oil
2 tablespoons baking soda
10 drops ylang ylang **or** Roman chamomile essential oil

1. Combine the sea salt, canola oil, and baking soda, then add the essential oil of your choice and blend well.
2. Moisten your skin. Rub small handfuls of the mixture on your arms and legs in circular motions. Wait a few minutes before rinsing.

Delegate or eliminate one 30-minute chore today. Perhaps family members can make their own lunch or do their own laundry. Or alternate shopping or cooking responsibilities with a friend. Be **CREATIVE** — any chore reduction frees up time to relax.

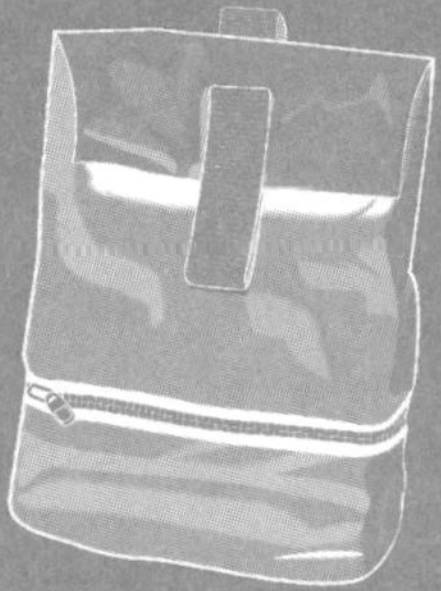

Peppermint Footbath

This footbath will soothe tired feet as it drains stress away.

1 gallon hot water
½ cup dried peppermint ***or***
4–8 drops peppermint essential oil

1. Fill a basin with steamy water and add either dried peppermint or peppermint essential oil.
2. Sit and submerge.

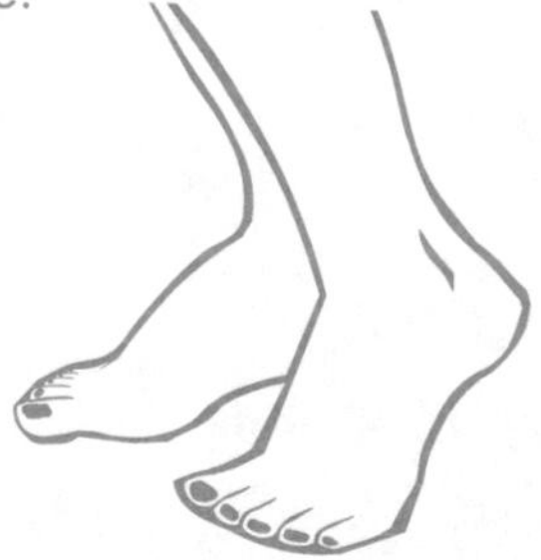

Picture That!

Keep your camera available and commit to snapping just one still photograph a day. Quiet down to focus while you glimpse life through a lens. Later, reflect as you page through your visual journal.

Beware of Stress-Causing Foods

The additive monosodium glutamate (MSG) can cause headaches and insomnia in sensitive individuals. Limit spicy or fatty foods, especially in the evening, as they can cause heartburn and disturb sleep.

"Don't just do something. Sit there."

Sylvia Boorstein

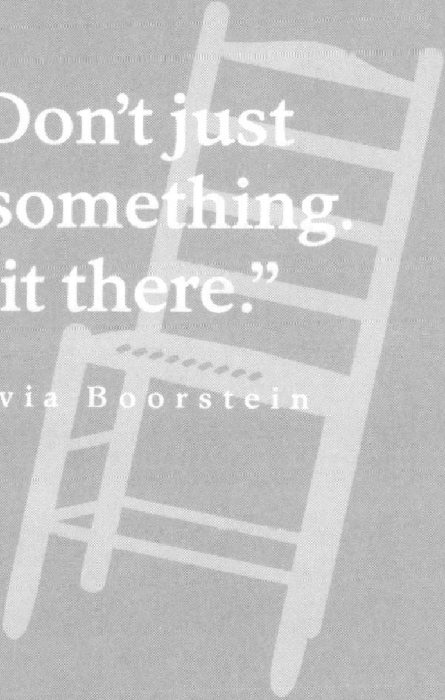

Make time this week to call your former neighbor who moved away, your college roommate, or an old friend you haven't spoken to in a while. Reminisce about the lazy days you once spent together.

Don't save that exciting bestseller for bedtime — you may not be able to put it down or stop thinking about it once you do. Reserve the half-hour before bed for an unsuspenseful novel or a collection of **INSPIRATIONAL** short stories.

Spas offer the **ULTIMATE** relaxation in idyllic settings. Your stay may include meditation, massage, hydrotherapy, yoga, hiking, salon services, and delicious, healthy meals. Or try a day spa as a reasonably priced alternative to full-service programs.

Communicate from the Heart

Clear and concise communication is freeing. Reflect upon what you think, how you feel, and what you want. Then, say what you mean, mean what you say, and don't say it mean.

Dim the Lights

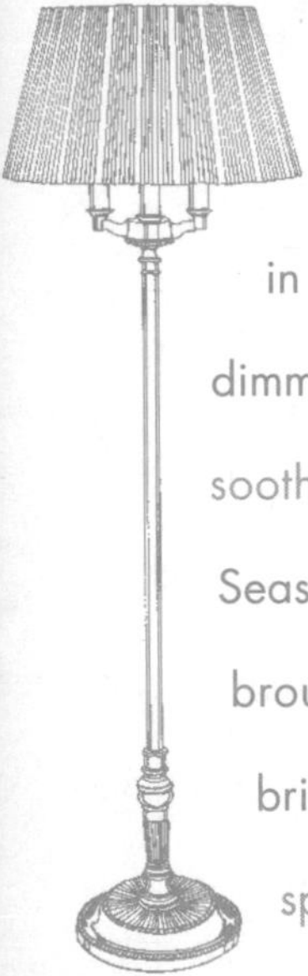

Bright lighting is important in the office, but soft lighting enhances relaxation in the bedroom or meditation space. Use dimmer switches to decrease energy use and soothe your mood. But if you suffer from Seasonal Affective Disorder, or depression brought on by winter's lower light level, brighten up with full-spectrum lights sold specifically to alleviate this problem.

A walk in the **WOODS** will improve your mood, provide you with a cardiovascular boost, and satisfy you visually. So put on some sturdy boots and grab your day pack to benefit from this great stress reliever.

“My special place
is a small brook
in a green glade,
a circle of quiet
from which there is
no visible sign of
human beings.
If I sit for

a while, then
my impatience,
crossness,
frustration are
indeed annihilated,
and my sense of
humor returns."

Madeleine L'Engle

Honey Mask

Stress exacerbates a number of chronic skin conditions. Try a honey mask to sweetly relax your face and avert possible problems. Honey is a natural moisturizer and has antioxidant, antibiotic, and antiviral properties.

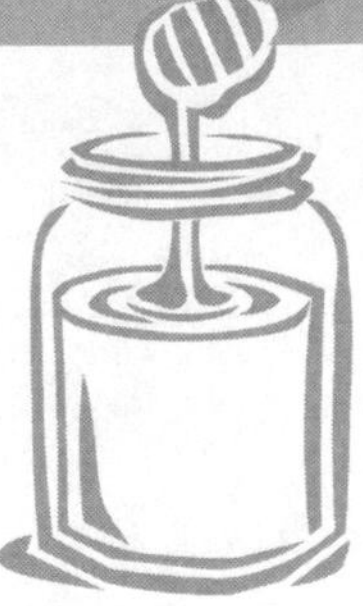

1. Pull your hair away from your face — pin it up or put it under a shower cap.
2. Apply a thin coat of honey to your entire face and neck.
3. Leave it on for 15 minutes while you lie down.
4. Rinse it off with tepid water.

Beware the ways of the "weekend warrior." Extra chores and active sports on those couple of days off often result in the pains of over-exertion. **SOOTHE** away muscle soreness with homeopathic arnica gel found in health food stores and natural pharmacies.

Leg Relaxer

Put your feet up — way up. Relax with the "legs-up-the-wall pose," a gentle modified yoga position.

1. Lie on the floor perpendicular to a wall with your buttocks as close to the wall as possible. Pad your buttocks with a light blanket.
2. Raise your legs and rest them along the wall.
3. Keep your head and shoulders on the floor. Rest your arms at your sides with your palms facing up.
4. Close your eyes and breathe slowly and deeply. Hold the pose for 5 minutes.
5. Bend your knees and roll onto your side to slowly release the pose.
6. Lie flat for another 2 minutes before standing up.

"Tomorrow is not promised, nor is today. So I choose to celebrate every day I'm alive by being present in it. Living in the present means letting go of the past and not waiting for the future."

Oprah Winfrey

Don't let your surroundings assault you. Blaring stereos, glaring lights, loud colors, and bold patterns attack your senses. Arrest demanding sights and distracting sounds with **CALM** alternatives. Reform your environment with soft music and soothing color.

Toning

Toning is a vocal technique that sustains a specific note or pitch. The vibrations of each sound resonate in different parts of your body. Try it: Sing a vowel sound — aaaahh, ooooo, eeeee — at any note. Experiment by lowering and raising your pitch. Choose one pitch and sustain the sound (taking extra breaths as needed) for 3 to 5 minutes.

Listen closely:
The signs of
serenity are often
more subtle than
the symptoms
of stress.

Fashion Your Own Fortune

Save those paper slips from fortune cookies with their fanciful forecasts, such as "You are destined for greatness" and "An around-the-world trip is in your future." Or write your own. How about "You will enjoy a peaceful and successful life"? Write it in your journal or tape a copy to the mirror you look in every morning.

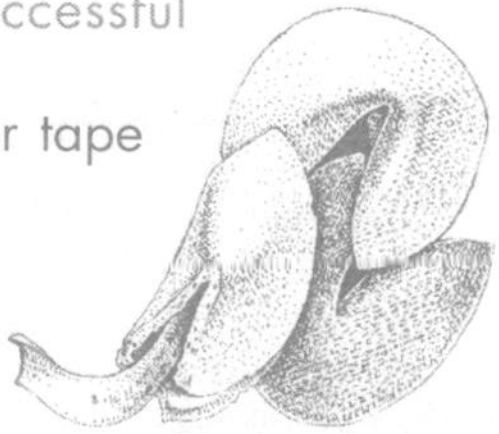

Allow yourself a **YAWN.** Since yawning has a bad reputation, you may want to wait until no one else is around. But yawning **FEELS GREAT.** It relieves tension, fatigue, and boredom. Just open your mouth wide and yawn. Stretch your arms over your head. After the first few, your yawns will roll out more easily.

It's a New Day

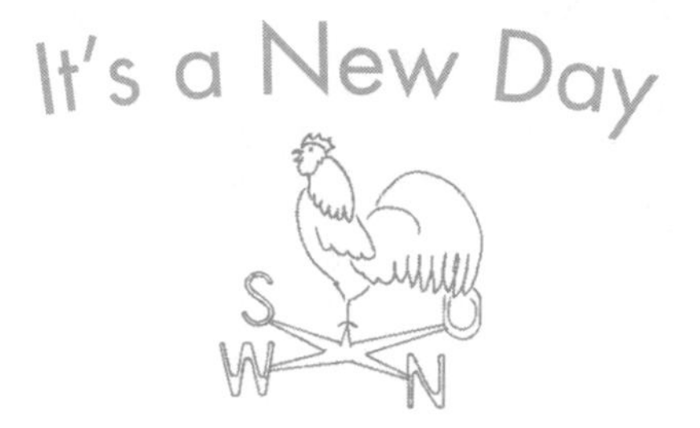

Delight in the dawning of a new day. Every day presents the promise of new perspectives and possibilities. It takes only a couple of minutes during your rushed morning routine to look out the window. Notice the brightening of the morning sky. Acknowledge the weather. Say thanks!

Frolic in
the fall foliage.
Playing in a pile of
autumn leaves
is one of the
best natural
tranquilizers.

Stock Up on Comfort Supplies

Fill a drawer with bubble bath, scented candles, a book of poetry, a few favorite photos, a small box of chocolates, and other personal indulgences. Save these goodies for a stressful day and let them refresh you when you need them the most.

Candle Meditation

1. Sit in a comfortable position. Light a candle on a small table in front of you at eye level.
2. Take a couple of deep breaths. Let the tension flow out of your body.
3. With your eyes half-open, gaze at the candle flame. Let the candle have all of your attention.
4. When your mind wanders, gently return to watching the flame.
5. After 5 minutes, close your eyes and look at the images behind your eyelids.
6. Slowly count to 20 and open your eyes.

Warm Hands, Warm Heart

Cold and calm are incompatible. You may feel especially chilled when afraid or stressed. To remedy this, run your hands and wrists under warm water for a few minutes. Gently pat your hands dry. Then wrap them around a mug full of steaming tea.

Bypass Beverages with a Buzz

To lessen anxiety and enhance your sleep, limit your consumption of coffee, black tea, and caffeinated soft drinks. Consuming 300 milligrams of caffeine — the equivalent of three cups of strong coffee or six cola drinks — at any time during a single day causes nighttime awakenings and disruption of the restorative REM sleep phase.

AFFIRMATIONS are positive, inspiring statements of qualities or outcomes that you desire, such as "I am filled with inner peace," "I have compassion for myself," or "I live in the present moment." Always state affirmations in the present, as if you already possess the quality. Repeat them to yourself throughout the day.

Don't Be the Best That You Can Be

Contrary to popular opinion, trying to be the best at everything doesn't lead to success; it is self-defeating. Perfectionism produces anxiety. Soften your standards and expectations on lower-priority items. You will be less frantic when you put your best efforts into activities of greater personal importance.

Hang Out in a Hammock

Let your body sink into relaxation while you float in an imaginary tropical paradise. Keep a glass of juice nearby, preferably garnished with a paper umbrella, and you may not want to return. City dwellers, please note: Although hammocks are best when hung between two shady trees, they can also be enjoyed indoors or on a balcony.

Don't allow **DINNER** to be disturbed by phone calls. Use your phone machine to screen calls. Lower the volume so the messages don't overpower the evening conversation.

TWINKLE TWINKLE

Your daily cares will slip away
as you scan the night sky. Even if you can't
identify the Big Dipper, on a clear night
you can't miss the tranquil twinkling of a star.

Studies show that listening to calm instrumental music before bed will help you nod off more quickly.

Prepare for Stress

When you're frazzled, your creativity and ability to self-nurture are diminished. So plan ahead. Make a list of 10 things that would gladden and console you. Include simple things, such as taking a walk, soaking your feet, calling a special friend, or anything that would make your life a little easier and your heart a little lighter. When you are feeling overburdened, take out your list. Don't think about it; just choose one thing and do it!

Purchase an **AROMATHERAPY** diffuser. When filled with your choice of essential oils, it will release small amounts of fragrance into the air. For a sedating scent, try a mixture of equal parts of Roman chamomile, neroli, and lavender.

Purchase a New Pillow

A pillow's capacity to keep your neck and spine in proper alignment is related to your sleeping position. Side sleepers benefit from a firm foam pillow. An additional pillow between your legs helps relieve pressure on your lower back and hips. Back sleepers rest better with a flatter pillow or one filled with soft down. Avoid sleeping on your stomach, if possible, since this position puts the most strain on your back.

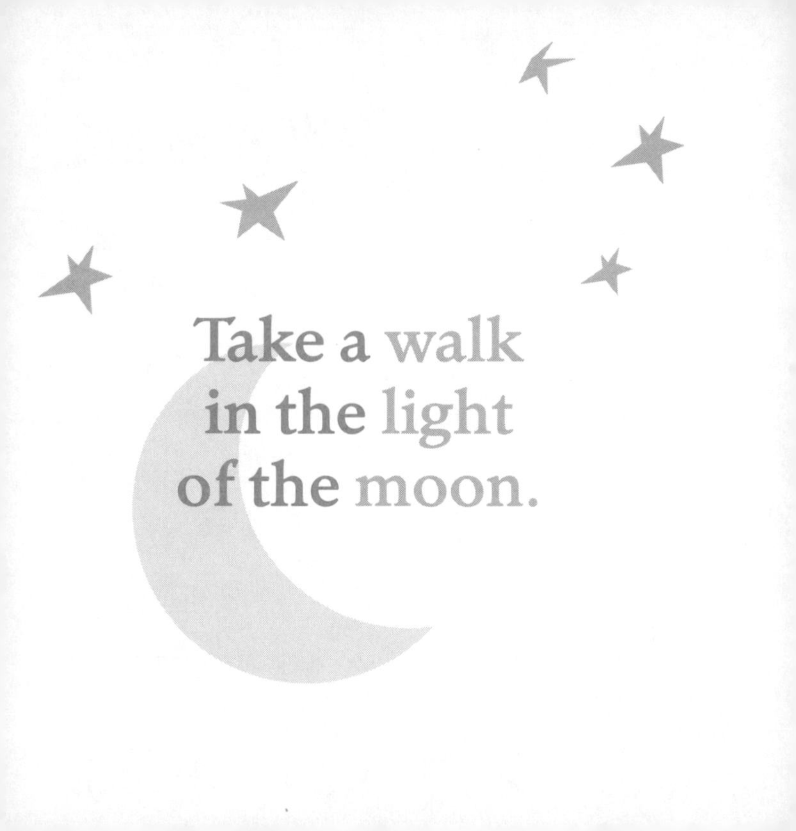
Take a walk
in the light
of the moon.

Cruise the Calming Cs

Be confident you have the capacity to cope. Commit to contemplation and you will create inner clarity and composure. Take comfort in comedy. Communicate your care and concern in compassionate action. This combination will keep you on course through the winds of change. Congratulations!

Before a stressful or difficult event, imagine yourself doing the task **WELL.** Picture yourself walking to the podium or swinging the bat. Internal imaginary practice increases self-confidence and improves your outcome. Using your **CREATIVE** center will help you feel calmer, too.

Hang some
wind chimes
by your window,
door, or porch.
Listen to the soft
music in the breeze.
Let the tinkling
lift your spirit.

Many cultures have used drums for healing and spiritual renewal. **DRUMMING** can connect you to a wordless inner space. Use your hand or a stick to beat a small drum. First, try to match the rhythm to your own heartbeat. Then experiment by speeding up the pace. Wind down by slowing the beat.

The Write Way

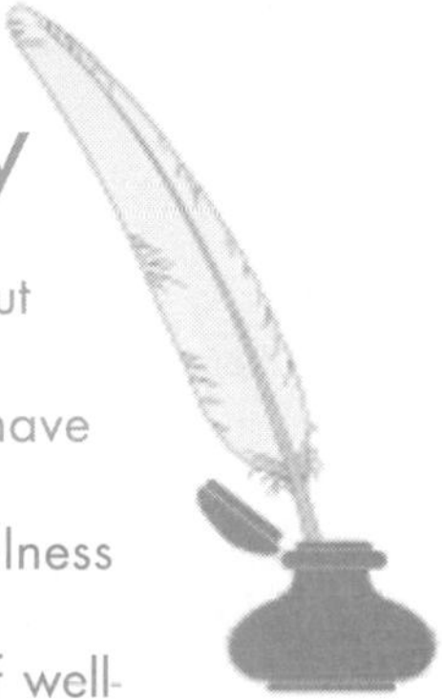

People who regularly write about their stressful experiences have fewer symptoms of chronic illness and develop a greater sense of well-being. Freely associate as you write, recording your innermost thoughts and feelings without censoring yourself.

Build a Personal Altar

Use it as a special place for reflection, prayer, and meditation. Choose a small side table or bench out of the way of family and company traffic. Cover it with a pretty cloth. Add a candle, figurines, stones, shells, photographs, fresh flowers, or other personally meaningful objects. Sit quietly in front of it for a few minutes every day.

Notice the **MAGICAL** quality of dusk. It is a time of in between. Distant hills reflect shimmering luminescence as the light dims, gradually fading. Take time to behold the beauty of nature's transitions.

Acquire an Affirmation Stone

There are many lovely painted rocks or porcelain markers available for purchase. Choose one with a trait or quality you want more of in your life, such as compassion, courage, acceptance, trust, beauty, or gratitude. Or make your own by painting your intention on a small, smooth stone. Place the stone on your kitchen counter, desk, or altar, or carry it with you as a daily reminder.

Share your space with other living things. Healthy potted plants and fish-filled aquariums create a calming effect in your home.

Develop **COOPERATIVE** calm in a massage class for couples. Or try partner yoga with videotaped instructions for stretching in tandem. Spend quality quiet time together and you'll appreciate a peaceful partnership.

Draw Stress Away

Expressive art therapists tell us that we can use art to go deeper than words can express, even if we have no artistic skill. Using the language of imagery reduces stress, helps us resolve personal conflicts, and gives voice to our inner messages. Purchase an art pad and some pastel chalks, crayons, or markers. Color your thoughts and emotions in shapes and images.

Savor a stunning sunset.

Listen to the sound
of water —
the rhythm of
ocean waves,
trickling waterfalls,
rushing streams,
raindrops, or an
indoor fountain.

NOURISH your relationship with your inner self by keeping a journal. Beginning journal writers often find beautiful blank books intimidating. Choose the journal equivalent of sweatpants — a spiral-bound or loose-leaf notebook is casual and comfortable. Invite your true self to hang out.

Turn Off Negative Thoughts

Thought stopping is a technique that can help you limit recurring unpleasant thoughts. Use it when your mind is like a tape recorder continually playing the same negative tune. When the distressing thought comes into your mind, say S-T-O-P. You can say it out loud. Picture yourself holding up a large stop sign. Or snap a rubber band on your wrist when the thought occurs.

Calming Position

This gentle position will help you slow down.

1. Sit in a straight-backed chair. Stretch your arms out in front with your palms touching.
2. Cross your hands over each other. Then flip them over so your palms are touching. Intertwine your fingers.
3. Fold your hands toward your heart until they are against your chest.
4. Stretch your legs out and cross your ankles.
5. Close your eyes and breathe slowly and deeply for 5 minutes.

Pin Up Peaceful Postcards

They'll provide instant art and atmosphere. You'll calm down when you see a sunflower, a small sailboat, or a lone soul on a rocky coastline. Choose a card with a serene landscape or a reproduction of a favorite painting to transform the mood of your workspace.

Choose a Comfortable Chair

Find the perfect one that rocks, revolves, or reclines. Add an afghan to wrap up with and a side table to hold a beverage. Read a book or take a snooze.

Lie down on the grass. Observe the sky on a calm day and notice how the clouds change shape. Feel the breeze brush your skin as nature softly breathes.

Set the Tone

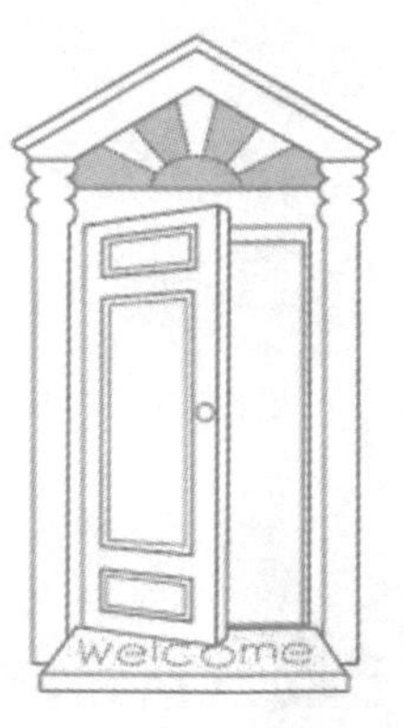

The threshold to your home should set a tone of calm and comfort. Provide a place to put down packages and to take off your outerwear. Small amenities, such as a tray for mail, hooks for keys, and an umbrella stand, will make the entryway even more inviting.

"Anything worth doing is worth doing slowly."

Colin Fletcher

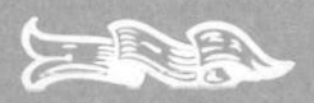

Schedule a weekly session with a **TRUSTED** friend. Take turns speaking for 15 minutes each. Talk about problems or vent about a situation. When you are the listener, be quiet, pay attention, and don't offer any solutions. It's very **SPECIAL** to listen and to be listened to; be rewarded by the give and take.

TranquiliTea

A cup of calming herbal tea provides the perfect antidote to a hectic day. There are many relaxing teas available without caffeine. You can make this special blend at home.

- 1 cup dried chamomile
- 1 cup dried lemon balm
- ½ cup dried catnip

1. Combine all ingredients and store in a tightly capped jar away from light and heat.
2. Use 1 teaspoon of the mixture for each cup of boiling water. Steep for 5 minutes.
3. Strain and add some honey, if desired.

Toast Your Tootsies

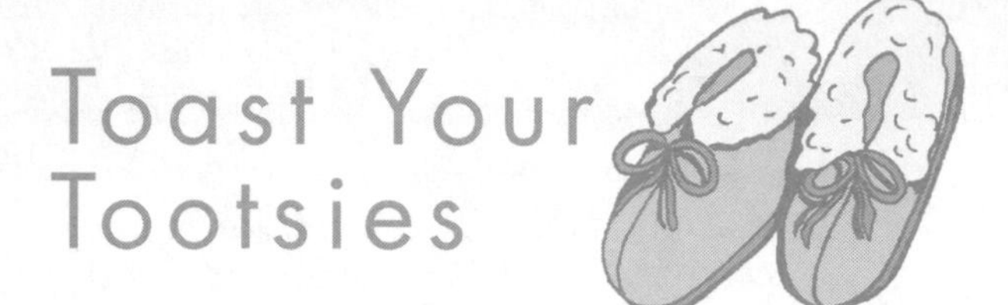

Warm feet are a natural sedative. Studies show that they help you fall asleep better than calming foods and supplements. Don some slippers or thick socks at bedtime or cuddle up with a hot-water bottle on your feet.

You can see the glass as half-full rather than half-empty. Remember that **PERSPECTIVE** is a habit. Tweak your long-standing negative patterns; people with optimistic outlooks live longer and healthier lives than do pessimists.

Having someone read to you is relaxing, and **AUDIOBOOKS** make it easy. Choose from the wide variety of bestsellers and classics available. It's a treat to listen to an author or noted actor read poetry, fiction, or biography. The tapes are great companions in the car or kitchen. Or listen to a soothing bedtime story before you go to sleep.

Bird Watching

It's no wonder that bird watching has been cited as one of the most relaxing hobbies. Early morning walks reward you with glimpses of flying and nesting birds in beautiful surroundings accompanied by the music of their sweet songs. Enhance your experience with a pair of binoculars and an identification book.

INDULGENCE

Bake a batch of your favorite cookies. To prolong the indulgence, eat a few warm cookies and share the extras with a friend.

The gardener's secret is that what appears to be hard work is also a salve for the soul.

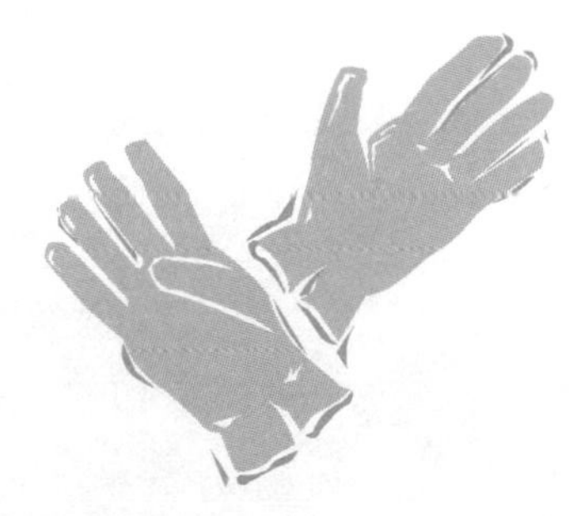

Strands of Serenity

Strands of beads have traditionally been used in contemplation and religious rituals. Make your own strand with pretty stones and ceramic beads. Spend some quiet time in a store bejeweled with sparkling display cases full of exotic gems, such as hematite, garnet, lapis, topaz, and rose quartz.

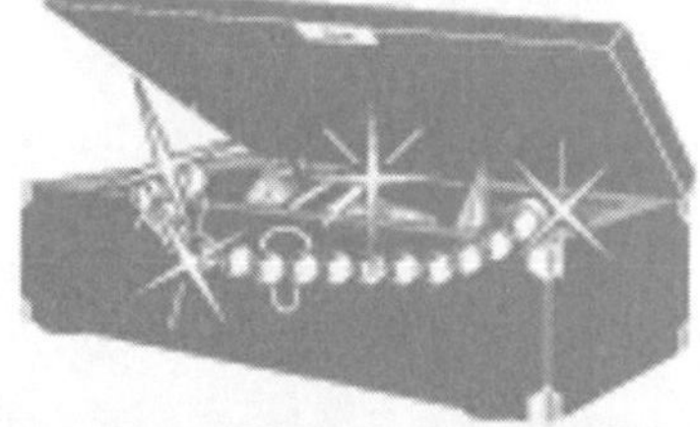

Ask yourself, "If I had **TODAY** to do over again, what would I do differently? What can I do tomorrow that will shape my day into a calmer and more satisfying one?" Choose one small change and by tomorrow's eve **RELISH** the rewards.

Time Management

Cut meaty tasks into bite-sized portions. When a project seems too large, break it down into many small steps. Compose a list of project-related activities that can be accomplished immediately. Write one page of that report, make one phone call, or outline a presentation. Keep yourself on schedule with weekly timelines and periodic rewards.

Write Your Own Prescription

People who write down their goals are more successful in realizing them than those who don't. Do you want to learn to meditate? Interested in taking a yoga class, going to a retreat, or changing your diet? List what you want to do and where and when you plan to do it. Include any special supplies or arrangements you need to accomplish your goal.

Take a needed midday **BREAK.** Don't skip lunch and don't grab a quick bite at your desk. Use this time to truly nourish yourself. Alternate between socializing and solitude. Some days, share your lunchtime with a friend. Other times, eat alone, preferably outdoors in a shady, **SECLUDED** spot.

Alternative Medicine

Try one of alternative medicine's many approaches to the treatment of stress and anxiety. Check out your community wellness center or complementary medicine department at a local hospital. Join the millions of Americans who are supplementing conventional treatment with acupuncture, chiropractic, homeopathy, and various forms of bodywork.

Take time
to smell the roses.
If there is none
in bloom,
purchase one
long-stemmed rose
in your
favorite color.

Place it where it will give you the most pleasure.

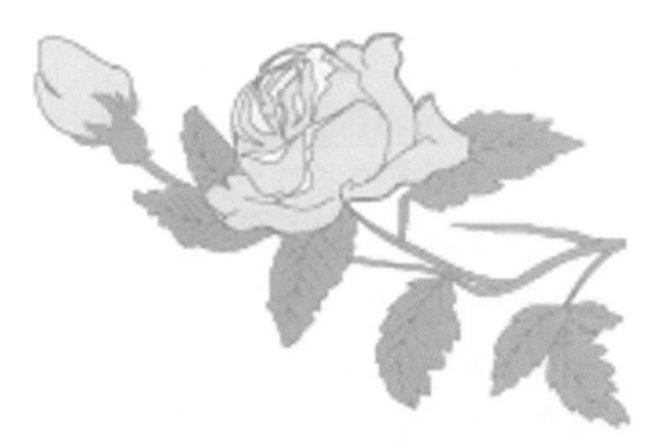

Color Me Calm

Different colors affect our moods. For clothing, choose complimentary colors that reflect your spirit. To create serene surroundings, decorate with light blues and greens.

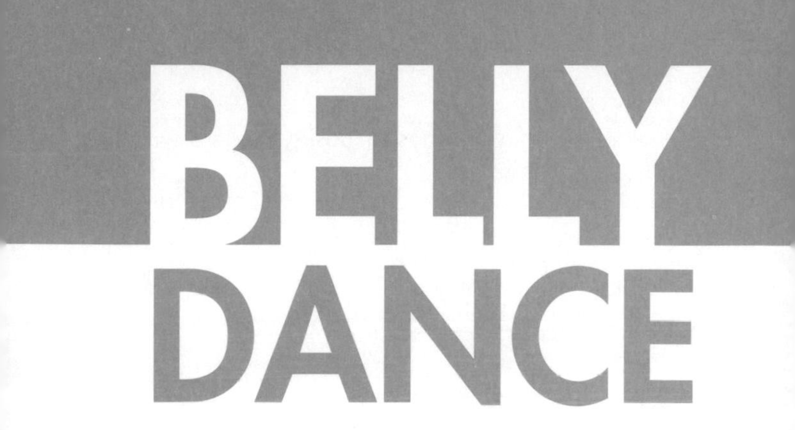

BELLY DANCE

The movements of this Middle Eastern art form are flowing and soft. You can swing your hips, waist, and arms to sensually release tension. Take a class or buy an instructional video.

Know Your Alternatives

There are two major ways to positively deal with stress. You can choose to change the stressful situation, such as by creating a quieter home or applying for a new job. Or you can work to change your physical and emotional responses to stress through exercise, meditation, and other means. Understanding your options is the first step to relaxation. List a few possibilities in each category before trying one.

"How beautiful it is to do nothing and rest afterwards."

Spanish Proverb

Share in communal song — join a choir, chant with a group, or conduct a sing-along.

Fill a jar or basket with some gel pens, stickers, rubber stamps, and various papers. Take a break and design some personal note cards. Or just **EXPERIMENT** with simple ways to express yourself.

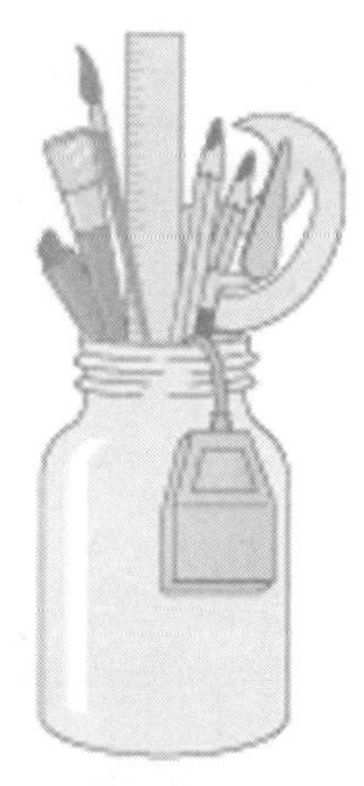

Share Your Bounty

Bring your neighbor a bunch of flowers or a batch of cookies. Share a good book with a co-worker. Tape a favorite show for a friend who is out of town. Seeing someone smile warms the heart and lifts the spirit.

Sit by the **FIRESIDE** and enjoy a cozy evening indoors. Curl up with a good book, share marshmallows and campfire tales, or simply watch the flames dance.

Take Three

Stop what you are doing for three minutes. Remember your three favorite vacation spots or visualize three of your preferred weekend pastimes. Pleasant recollections instill calm. Return to your task with a new perspective.

Cleansing Breath

Deep breathing is the most efficient way to return to a steady state.

1. Inhale through your nose for a count of 4. Hold for a count of 1.
2. Exhale for 8 counts — let your breath out audibly through puckered lips as if you are blowing out a candle. Then hold for a count of 4.
3. Repeat several times.

Visualize that you are breathing in quiet and stillness and breathing out noise and tension.

Walk the simple path to serenity. Find a **LABYRINTH** in your area or schedule a visit to one in another community. Experience peaceful introspection and increased intuition during this walking meditation. You'll find the benefits are truly amazing.

Keep a small notebook for inspiration. Fill it with favorite quotes and words of quiet wisdom. Reap its rewards on a stressful day.

Recite Your ABCs

When you are confronted with a stressful situation, it is helpful to pause before you act.

1. **A**cknowledge the situation. Summarize it to yourself internally or out loud to another person.
2. **B**reathe deeply and slowly.
3. **C**onsider your options, then choose your direction.

Pull some weeds and trim some shrubs. Both you and your yard will benefit.

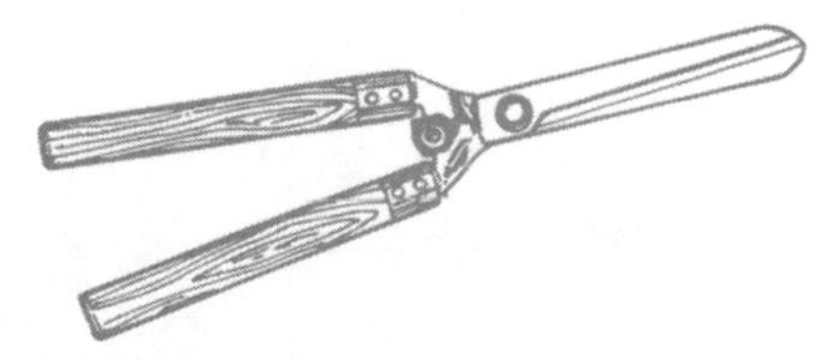

Comfort Foods

Do chocolate pudding, chicken soup, macaroni and cheese, or other childhood favorites remind you of easier times? Which foods did you eat when you were sick or feeling down? Keep some of those soothing foods on hand and be nourished by the memories.

Travel an inner **JOURNEY** with a journal. Daily entries will help you identify your feelings and clarify your choices. Giving voice to your inner thoughts lets your heart and soul catch your attention. Date all entries. Save and keep your journals in a private place.

Open the **WINDOW** and let the outdoors in. Stale, stagnant air stresses the body. Soothe your senses with nature's sights, smells, and sounds even if you don't have time to go outside. If the weather is really bad, just sit and calmly look out the window for a few minutes.

White Light Meditation

Try this meditation technique for a sense of peaceful protection.

1. Sit comfortably in a chair or cross-legged on the floor.
2. Breathe deeply and fully.
3. Visualize a shimmering light shining on you from above.
4. Picture this light forming an opaque shield around your entire body.
5. Internally affirm, "I am sheltered. I am protected. I am safe and secure."

Young children live only in the present moment. Talk with a child, listen to a child, read to a child, and play with a child. See the world from a child's point of view.

Throw Something Away

Discard items not working, clothes not worn, and gadgets not used. Donate items that others can put to better use. Recycling is good for the soul.

Change Your Response to Stress

When faced with a crisis, we often resort to "fight or flight" responses. We get defensive, argue, or make a hasty, angry retreat. Instead, choose to "tend and befriend," which is a healthier response. Those who relate to others and talk with supportive friends weather a crisis more satisfactorily.

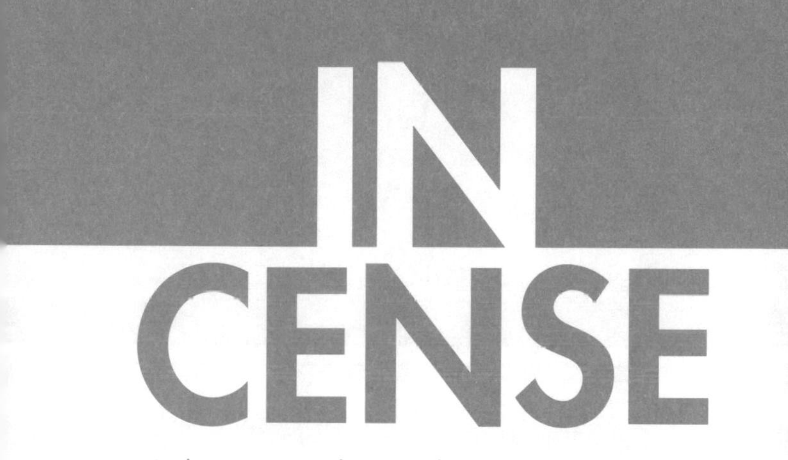

Light incense to bring calm to your space. Let it smoke during a quiet period of daily reflection. As you learn to associate calm with its scent, the benefits will increase over time.

Have a Personal Pajama Party

Stay indoors on a Saturday or Sunday. Loll around until the after-noon in your favorite pajamas, an oversized bathrobe, some colorful socks, and slippers.

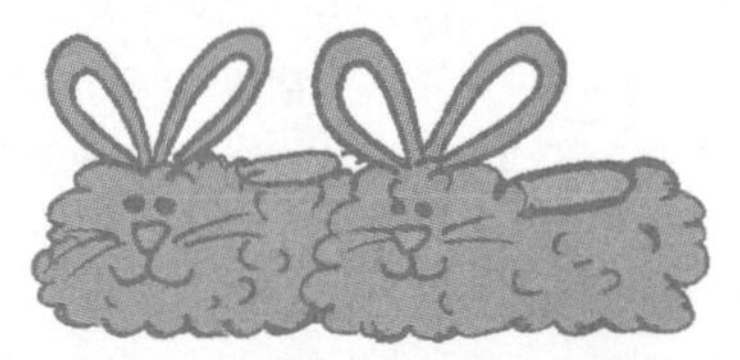

Get a colorful perspective through a **KALEIDOSCOPE.** It's a wonderfully relaxing way to view the world. Hold one of these mirrored tubes up to the light and turn it gently to see the colorful patterns change.

In this e-mail era, pen a personal note to a long-lost friend, a distant relative, or a college student away from home. Writing by hand gives you a chance to **REFLECT.** Share your stories and some good wishes.

Pace Yourself

When faced with a large project, don't start with a spurt like a sprinter. And don't expect to sustain the same pace throughout the task. To maintain momentum, stride like a marathon runner. Allow yourself cycles of energy and achievement, slowing and quickening for different segments. Remember to rest after you've crossed the finish line.

BRAIN STORM

When stressed, you may feel stuck in your situation and unable to see options. Enlist help from friends and family to brainstorm creative ideas and alternatives.

Stop, Look, and Listen

Diffuse a stressful situation "sense-ably." Close your mouth and open your ears and eyes. Your initial tendency may be to jump in and defend. But if you watch and listen to the other person first, your response will be more balanced.

“When one is a
stranger to oneself,
then one is estranged
from others, too.

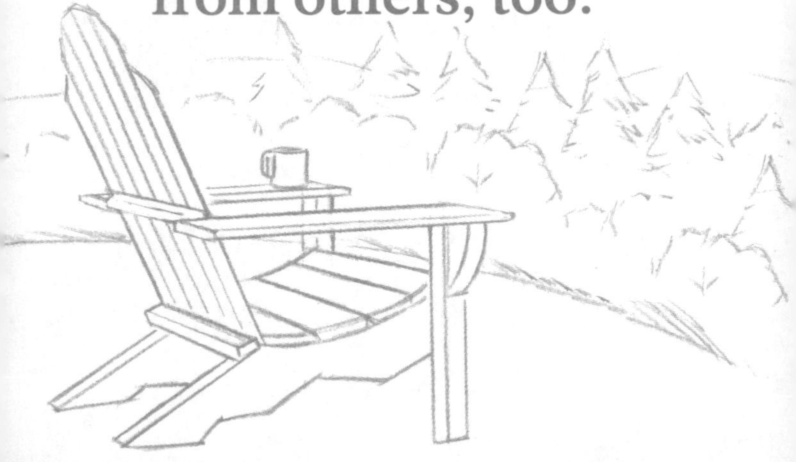

Only when one is connected to one's core is one connected to others. The core, the inner spring, can best be refound through solitude."

Anne Morrow Lindbergh

Heed your
heart
as well as your
head.

❤

Create a Collage

Collect words and images cut from magazines and catalogs. Combine them with decorated papers, string, stamps, and other pleasing items. Allow your unconscious to guide your artistic assemblage.

Rejoice in Resolution

Don't call attention to your own bloopers. Often, we put the spotlight on our defects and blunders. We make them larger than life. Next time you make a mistake, calmly assess the damage, make possible corrections, and then move on. Revisit the concern at the end of the day and decide whether you need to do anything more. Then rejoice in your resolution.

Every evening, list five things that happened that day for which you are grateful.

Stand Up and Stretch

1. Stand with your feet hip-width apart.
2. Interlace your fingers and raise your hands above your head with your palms facing upward.
3. Inhale and stretch up toward the sky.
4. Exhale and lean gently to the left (hands at "11 o'clock").
5. Inhale, return to center, and again stretch upward.
6. Exhale and lean gently to the right (hands at "1 o'clock").
7. Inhale, return to center, and stretch upward.
8. Exhale and release your arms.

Replenish Your Reserves

Take a trip to a museum, arboretum, or planetarium. Sign up for a walking tour of neighborhood architectural styles. Try something new or rekindle an old interest.

Designate today as your personal **TOUCH** day. To eliminate tension, stretch your sense of touch. Ask yourself these three questions: Which sensations delight me? Which textures relax me? What might I feel today?

"Have nothing
in your houses
that you do not
know to be useful,
or believe
to be beautiful."

William Morris

Pause for Perspective

Lie on your back on a soft surface with your legs on the floor and your feet 6 to 8 inches apart. Place your hands by your sides, palms up. Take slow, deep breaths. Release your tension into the ground. Just 3 to 5 minutes in this pose could change your outlook for the day.

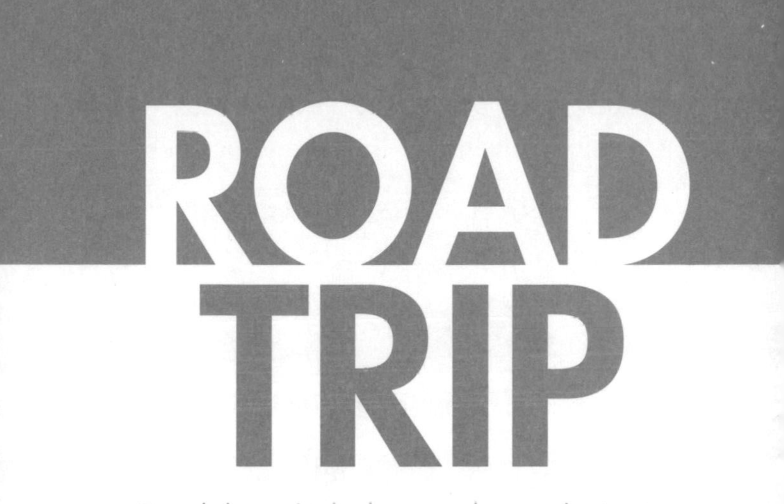

Travel down the highway without a destination. Plan a few days for exploration and sight-seeing.

Lower Back Stretch

1. Lie on your back. Keep your knees together and raise them to your chest.
2. Wrap your arms around your legs. Gently hug your knees to your chest while keeping your lower back flat on the floor.
3. Raise your head to your knees.
4. Hold for 10 seconds and then relax. Repeat twice.

Activate the pressure points of your hands to **RELEASE** stress. Clasp your hands together. Press and release your interlocked fingers five times, putting pressure at the base of each finger.

"A spiritual retreat is medicine for soul starvation. The retreat is not an end in itself; it is simply a method to help us slow down and stop.

Through silence,
solitary practice,
and simple living,
we begin to
fill the empty
reservoir."

David A. Cooper

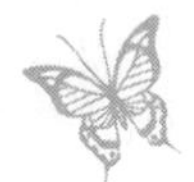

Herbal Sleep Pillows

Sew or purchase an herbal sleep pillow made to fit between your pillowcase and pillow. Its sedative scent will be released each time you turn your head during the night. Try a combination of dried lavender, rose petals, hops, chamomile, and lemon balm.

Consider an overnight stay at a retreat center. An inexpensive **GETAWAY** provides you with basic room and board. The long periods of quiet and reduced responsibilities will help you reclaim your spiritual center.

Guided Imagery

Imagine yourself in a field of wildflowers. Picture a Monet canvas of many colors, shapes, and textures. Walk across the vibrant meadow with the sun gleaming behind you. Stay as long as you wish in this safe and serene spot.

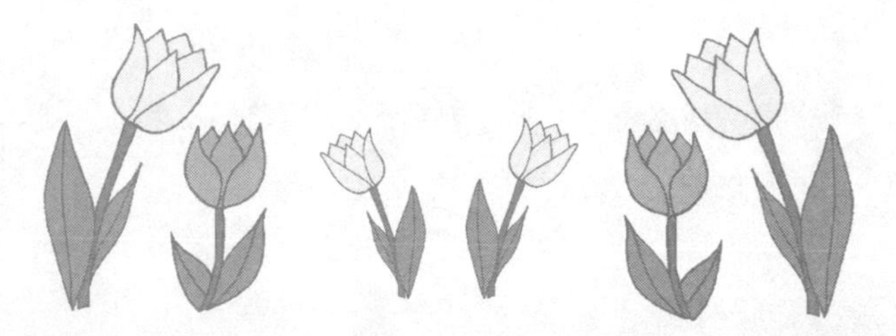

Leg Stretch

1. Sit on the floor with your legs open as wide as is comfortable.
2. Turn your torso toward your left foot. Bend from the waist and keep your chin parallel with the ground as you gently stretch forward. Hold but don't strain.
3. Release, then repeat twice.
4. Repeat on your right side.

Yesterday's Toys

Skip a Slinky down the stairs, "walk the dog" with a yo-yo, or count the times you can hit the ball on its attached wooden paddle.

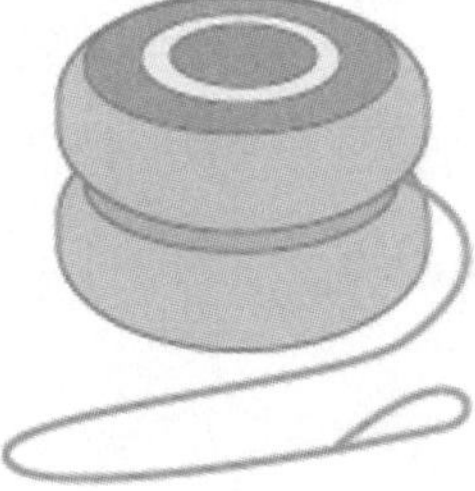

GREEN HOUSE

These structures provide the perfect environment for buds and blooms. Stroll through the plant-filled aisles and you'll flourish right along with the flowers.

Face Massage

A face massage helps relieve stress and soothe stuffed sinuses.

1. With the index and middle fingers of each hand, gently rub around your eyes from the inner corners to the outer corners.
2. Using your thumbs, start at the bridge of your nose and massage across the line of your eyebrows.
3. Apply pressure to the sensitive points in the middle of your eyebrows.
4. Rub down the bridge of your nose with your index and middle fingers.
5. With gentle pressure, sweep across your cheek bones and out toward your ears.

Enjoy community entertainment at a street fair or festival. Area colleges also have fun events open to the public. Check for listings in local newspapers.

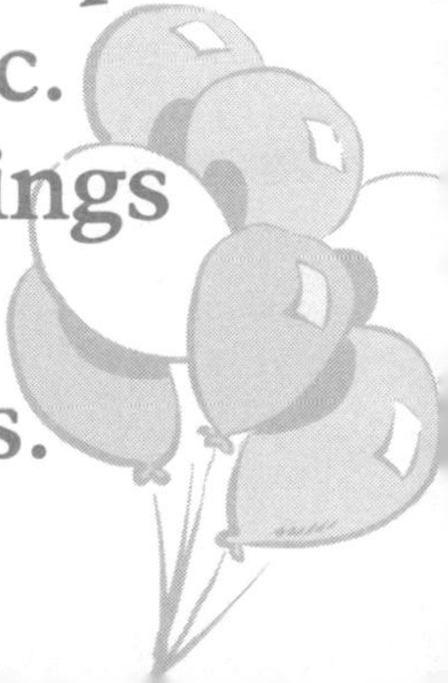

Head, Neck, and Shoulder Stretch

The head, neck, and shoulders form a "tension triangle." Try this stretch to release stress.

1. Sit in a cross-legged position or in a comfortable chair with your feet on the floor. Place your hands on your knees.
2. Drop your head to your chest.
3. Inhale and slowly rotate your head toward your right ear. Don't tip your head back.
4. Hold, exhale, and slowly return to an upright position.
5. Repeat on your left side.

Sit by the water's edge. Skip stones across a pond. Dip your toes in the lake. Listen to the surf break.

Relive Romance

A recent medical study indicates that romantic fantasies lessen pain and promote relaxation. When participants fantasized or recalled romantic times spent with a special someone, their anxiety levels dropped.

Blow Bubbles

Buy a bottle of magical bubble-making liquid. Dip in the bubble wand and whoosh to release the rainbow orbs. Imagine your cares floating away with the vanishing bubbles.

Stop doing and start being. Today, see how long you can do nothing.

Toe Twister Stretch

1. Sit comfortably in a chair. Rest your right foot on your left knee.
2. Grasp your right foot in your right hand with your thumb across the instep on the underside of your foot. Your other four fingers should be on the top of your foot.
3. Place your left hand higher up your foot next to your right hand with your thumbs parallel.
4. Twist the top of your foot toward you with your left hand. Use your right hand to keep your foot steady.
5. Move both hands up your foot in half-inch increments and continue the twisting motion.
6. Repeat on your left foot.

Camp Out

Close a day of active outdoor activity with star watching and singing around the campfire. Appreciate the fresh air and night sounds from the cocoon of calm inside your tent.

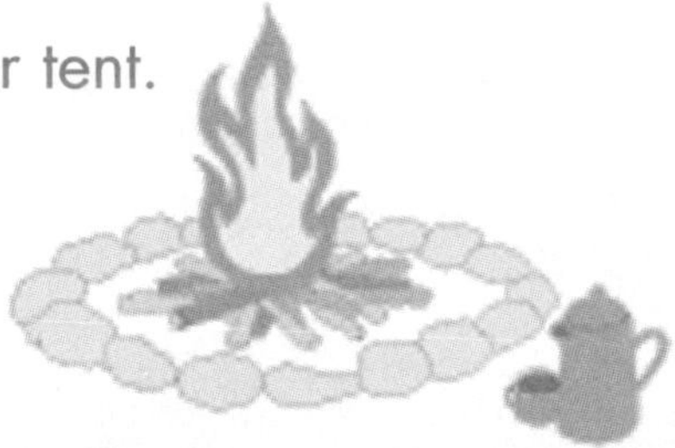

Go **OUTDOORS** and play catch. Or bounce, hop, and roll on inflatable jumbo gym balls. A bad-weather alternative is indoor catch, played with pairs of rolled-up socks. Just make sure the breakables are out of the way.

"Life is a good teacher and a good friend."

Pema Chodron

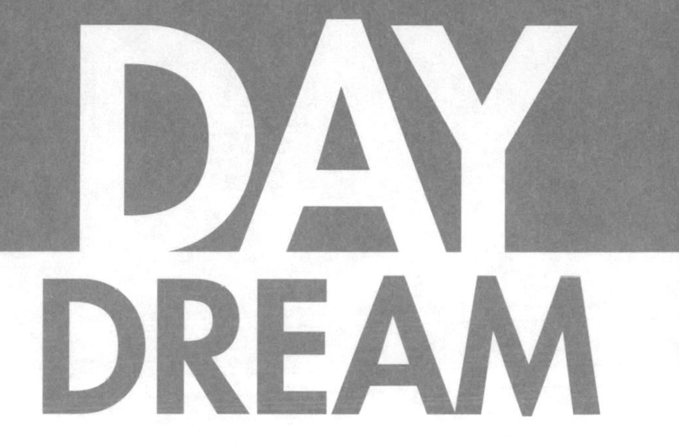

Daydreaming is not a waste of time. Honor these relaxing reveries. If you pay attention to your imaginative visions, you'll learn more about what your heart really wants.

Go for a
Sunday drive.
Cruise the country-
side, stopping
at farm stands and
flea markets.

Make Music

Play a tune on the piano. Strum a song on the guitar. For a melodic meditation, musicians recommend performing an old favorite piece rather than a new challenging one.

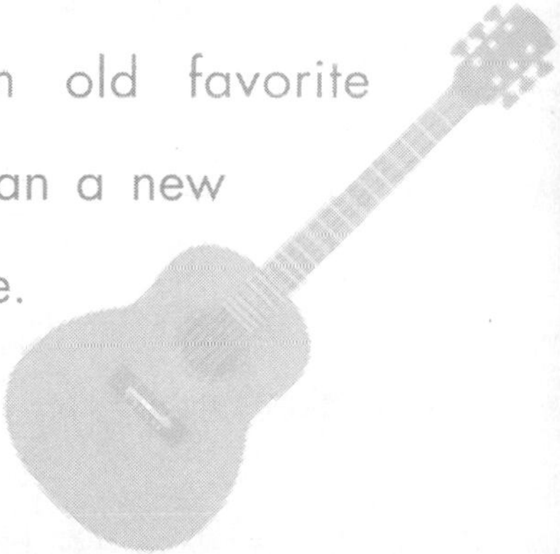

Arm Rolls

Arm rolls increase circulation and flexibility while releasing tension from your upper body.

1. Stretch your arms out to your sides with your palms facing down and your elbows straight. Keep your shoulders down.
2. Take a few calming breaths.
3. Rotate your arms in small circles. Slowly increase to larger circles.
4. Make 5 to 10 circles in each direction.

Seasonal Meditation

Imagine bright flower borders, trees bending in the breeze, and watermelon seeds at a summer picnic. Next, visit in your mind's eye the harvesting of crops and the colors of a changing autumn. Follow this with icy visions of sugarplum fairies, fireplaces, hot chocolate, and sleds. End with spring rain, birdsong, and longer days. Personalize your visualization with your own favorite tastes, smells, and sounds from each season.

Join a Club

Social connections strengthen your mind, body, and spirit. Try a bowling league, book club, hiking group, or political committee.

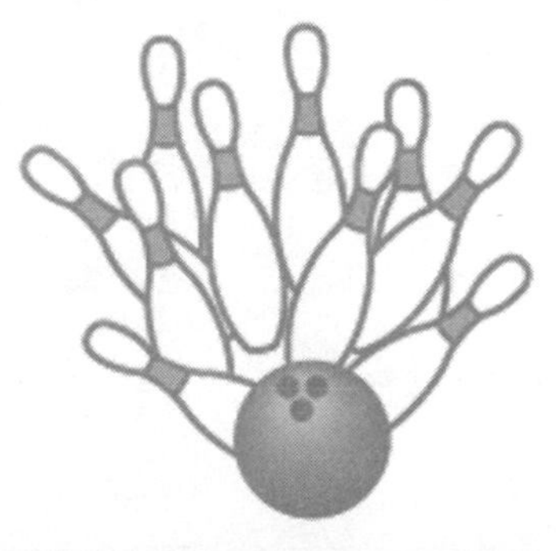

Steam Facial

Soothe stress with a cleansing and calming steam facial.

1. Put a handful of dried chamomile and calendula flowers in a large ceramic bowl.
2. Pour in boiling water until the bowl is three-quarters full.
3. Make a tent with a towel over your head and the bowl.
4. Savor the wafting scents. Take care not to burn yourself.

Fruit Salad

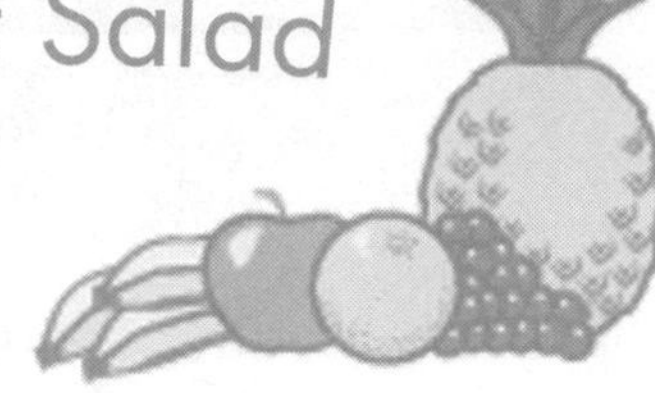

Mindfully prepare this simple meal.

First, go to the farm stand or grocer and choose a variety of ripe fruit. In your kitchen, wash, peel, and slowly chop your selections. Focus on the feel and fragrance of each fruit. Decorate with raisins, sunflower seeds, coconut, and yogurt. Eat the salad slowly to appreciate the distinctive yet blended flavors.

Studies by university researchers show that "prophylactic napping," or **NAPPING** in advance of a long stretch of activity, can improve one's memory, mood, judgment, and creativity. Prepare for an upcoming meeting with a pre-presentation snooze.

Indulge in intimacy.
Take time to
converse
meaningfully
and touch gently.

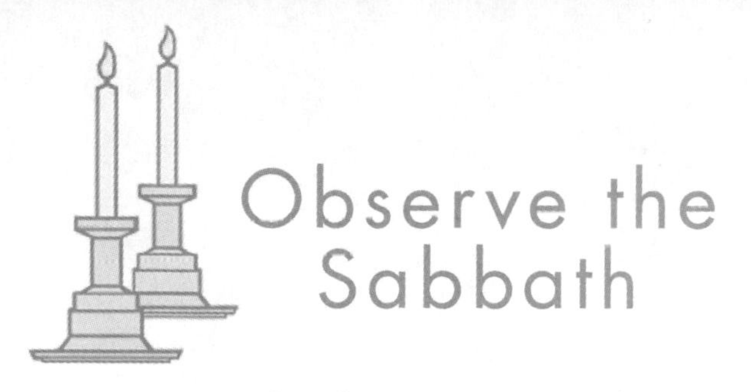

Observe the Sabbath

Organized religions remind us to take a break from our regular activity. Designate your own personal day of rest. Reserve a few hours a week for quiet reflection, meditation, or sharing a meal with others.

Designate today as your personal **SOUND** day. To relieve the symptoms of stress, stretch your sense of hearing. Ask yourself these three questions: Which sounds delight me? Which sounds relax me? What might I hear today?

Find a New Hobby

Spend your leisure time researching your family tree, collecting teapots or rare books, or working on the sports car that you drive only in the summer. A personal part-time pleasure will add a relaxing dimension to your busy life.

Complete These Sentences

1. One of the most positive traits I have is

   ____

   ____.

2. The two things I do best are ____________________

   ____ and

   ____.

3. I have a talent for ____________________________

   ____

   ____.

Prominently post your answers in your personal space. Let them serve as daily reminders of your strengths and positive attributes.

"Simple pleasures are the best."

Bobby McFerrin

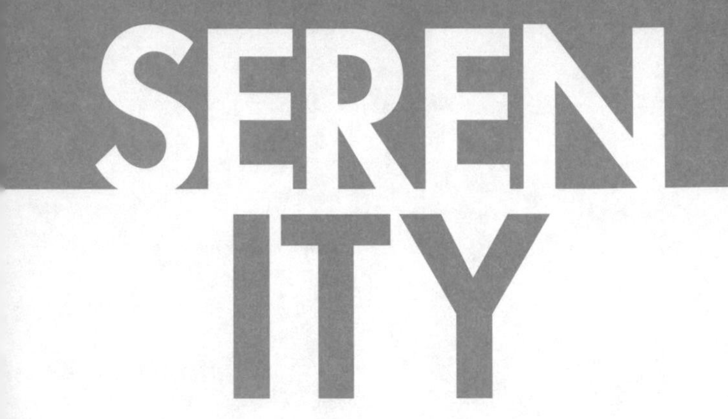

When traveling, stash a small herb-filled sachet in your carry-on luggage. It will soothe you during plane trips and sweeten nights spent in stuffy hotel rooms.

Relaxing Room Spray

Mist your bedroom with one of these relaxing room sprays.

- 6 ounces distilled water
- 20 drops total of bergamot, sandalwood, and clary sage essential oils ***or***
- 20 drops total of lavender, ylang ylang, and patchouli essential oils ***or***
- 20 drops total of lavender, marjoram, and mandarin essential oils

1. Add the water to one of the essential oil combinations.
2. Shake well before each use and don't spray on furniture.

Although any spray bottle will do, the mixture looks great in a cobalt-blue glass atomizer.

“Meditation can release certain facets of your mind that usually remain in the background. They reside in every person’s mind but they come out only when they are welcomed with quietness, awareness, and observation. They are creativity and intuition."

American Yoga Association

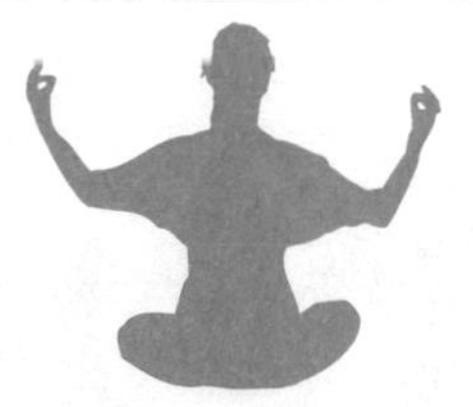

Peel an **ORANGE** slowly and deliberately. Let the aroma transport you. Enjoy eating the sections just as they are or dip them, fondue style, into melted chocolate.

Rip Stress to Shreds

Don't let stress rip you apart; instead, tear it up. Here's a safe way to physically release tension. Rip out a few pages of an old newspaper and ball them up. Throw them across the room. Shred pages into small pieces or tear a section of the paper in half and then in half again. When you're done, your recovery from stress will be newsworthy.

Designate today as your personal **TASTE** day. Let go of bitterness and strife by stretching your sense of taste. Ask yourself these three questions: Which flavors delight me? Which flavors relax me? What might I taste today?

Whistle
a happy
tune.

Make Snow Angels

Lie down flat on your back in the snow. Spread your arms up and down to make your wings.

"The present moment is where life can be found, and if you don't arrive there, you miss your appointment with life. You don't have to run anymore. Breathing in, we say, 'I have arrived.' Breathing out, we say, 'I am home.'"

Thich Nhat Hanh

HEED the message "Mending is better than ending." This old adage still has merit. Don't throw away that torn shirt or skirt in need of a hem. Keep a basket of sewing supplies and small items that need fixing by a comfy chair. Background music will help you **MUSE** while you mend.

Row, Row, Row Your Boat

Let your cares float away during a day on the water. Cruise the currents in a small, nonmotorized boat. Canoeing is calming and sailing is serene.

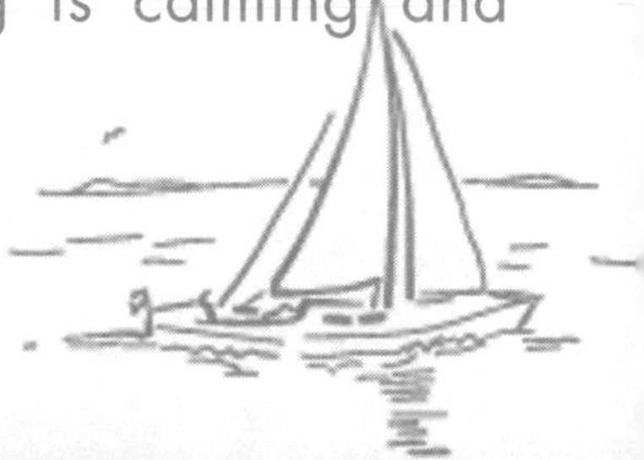

"May you have
warm words
on a cold evening,
a full moon
on a dark night, and
the road downhill
all the way
to your door."

Mary Engelbreit

Stress-Relief Pose

This simple relaxation posture is great for a midafternoon break. It can be done almost anywhere — at home, while you are traveling, or in your office with the door closed.

1. Lie down on your stomach. (This is best done on the floor with some padding, not on a bed.)
2. Place your arms by your sides with your palms facing up. Lean your head to one side, with your cheek to the floor.
3. Take five slow deep breaths. Release, and then relax.
4. Turn your head to the other side and repeat. Let the tension flow out of you.
5. To get up, roll over on your side and push up with your arms.

Meander

Take a stroll
without a purpose
or a
destination.

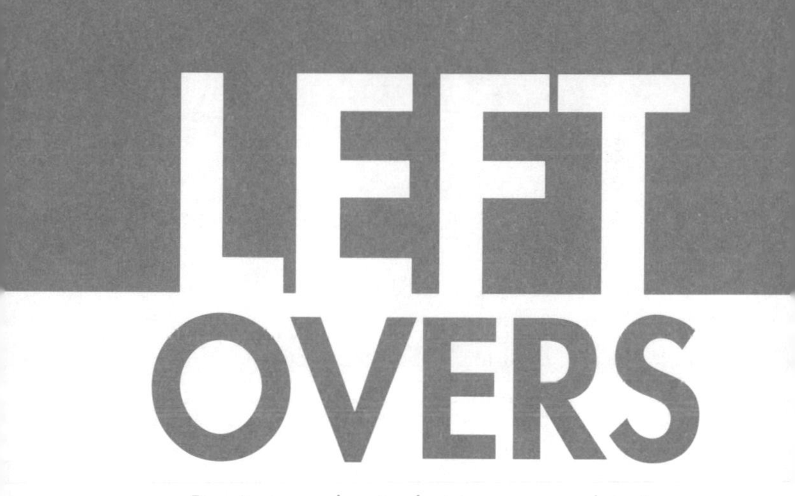

Don't stew about what to eat on a hectic weeknight. When cooking a large meal on the weekend, prepare extra portions to freeze. Warm up the leftovers when needed.

Be Prepared

When shopping, purchase duplicates of the items that you use frequently. Bring extra pantyhose, lozenges, or aspirin to the office. Keep sample-sized soap and toothpaste packed in your travel kit. And to avoid those last-minute trips to the store, buy extra batteries, candles, matches, and school and office supplies.

Start a "Blue Day" File

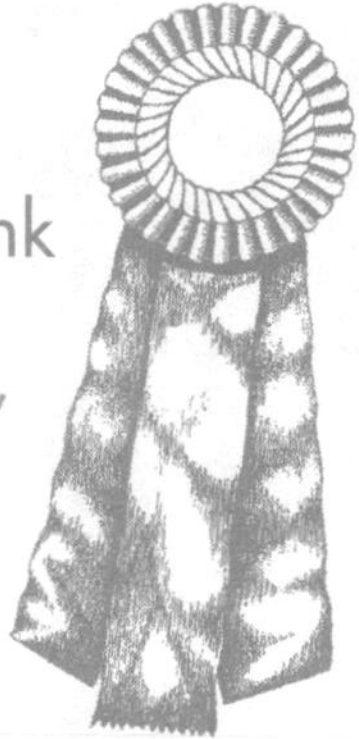

Fill a file with copies of thank you notes, moving tributes, honors, and awards that you've received. When skies are gray, reread this pile of special missives. It's great medicine for melancholy.

SNAP SHOTS

Leaf through a photo album for a close-up of your past. Relax alone with these remembrances or share them with someone as you view old snapshots.

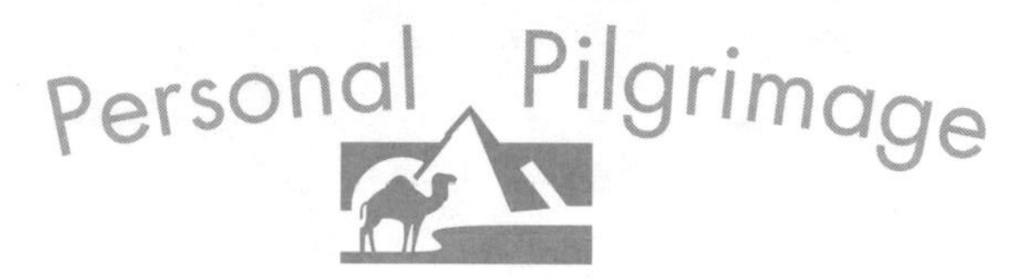

Design a personal pilgrimage for internal peace. Even if you can't afford to trek in Nepal or visit the power spots of Sedona, you'll benefit from planning an imaginary trip to a sacred place. Choose an area you've always dreamed of visiting. Learn more about it. Collect some travel brochures. Speak to people who have been there. Find fulfillment in your fantasy — but you can also start saving loose change for the future possibility.

Cooperation

Learn to work and play well with others. Give family members and colleagues credit for their contributions. Be generous with your comfort and support. You'll create a win-win situation that lessens conflict. Cooperative efforts score high on the satisfaction scale.

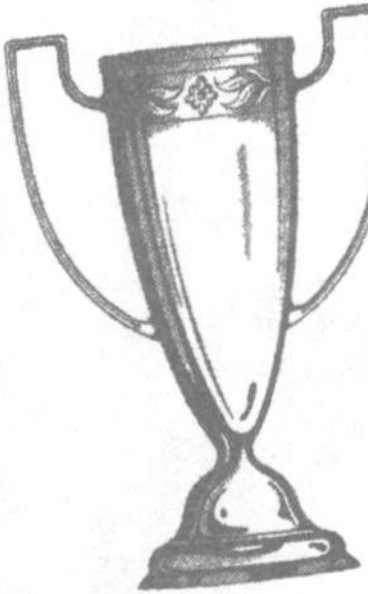

"The window to
the spirit
is the silent spaces
between
our thoughts."

Deepak Chopra

Spend a Day at the Beach

Surf the waves. Read a romance or mystery novel under the umbrella. Contemplatively comb the beach for shells. Build a sand castle.

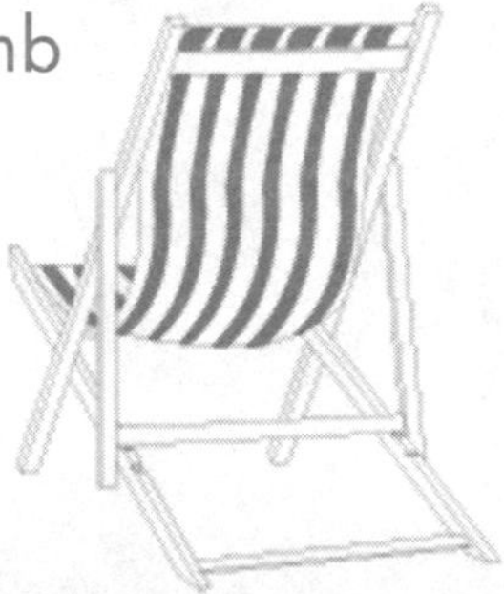

Listen
for the voice
of your inner
wisdom.

Awaken Slowly

Allow yourself to gradually wake up and become aware of the world around you. Don't jump out of bed. Open your eyes, slowly uncurl, and savor the state of mind between dreaming and alertness. Stretch and smile.

UN PLUGGED

Turn off the palm pilot, computer, answering machine, fax, beeper, and cellular phone. Make believe you've been cast off on a tropical island. Be technology-free for one day.

Hum a lullaby
to a little one
while swaying in a
rocking chair.
This is especially
relaxing with a
grandchild or a
neighbor's newborn.

Choose Low-Maintenance Objects

Surround yourself with items that don't demand a lot of extra care. Don't purchase clothes that require dry cleaning or plants that need daily attention. Lessen the demands on your time and energy.

Eat like a European

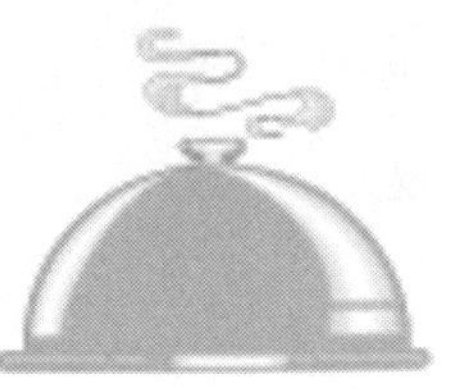

Dining in France means lingering for hours, enjoying conversation and numerous small courses. Reserve one evening a week to leisurely enjoy a traditional meal.

"We need
time to dream,
time to remember,
and time to
reach the infinite,
time to be."

Gladys Taber

Buy Local Produce

Shop at the farmers' market. Purchase local produce, preferably grown organically, from the proud farmer who planted and harvested it. This true soul food will nourish your body and your spirit.

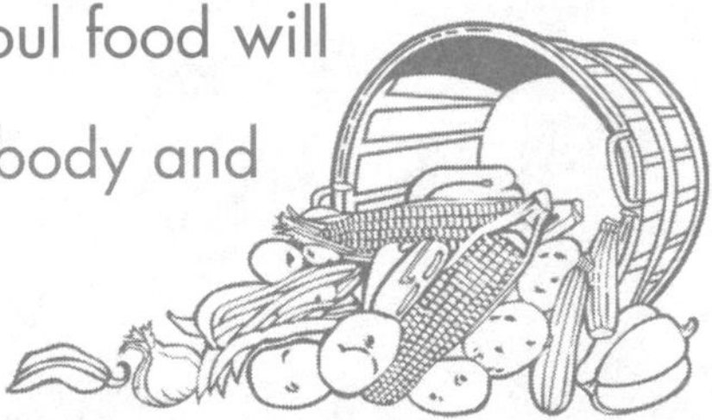

Serenity Position

A moment or two of stillness in this simple position will calm you down.

1. Sit on the floor with the soles of your feet together.
2. Clasp your hands around your feet and pull your heels as close to your body as possible.
3. Gently press your knees toward the floor. Take a few deep breaths.
4. Release your feet and relax.
5. Repeat.

Everyone needs
a good cry.
Whether watching
a sad movie or
mourning a loss,
don't hold back
your tears.

Wait to Answer the Phone

Curb the urge to jump at the phone's insistent ringing. Instead, think of the telephone as a bell sounding the call for inner balance. Take deep and slow breaths while you wait until the second or third ring. Pick up slowly and say hello.

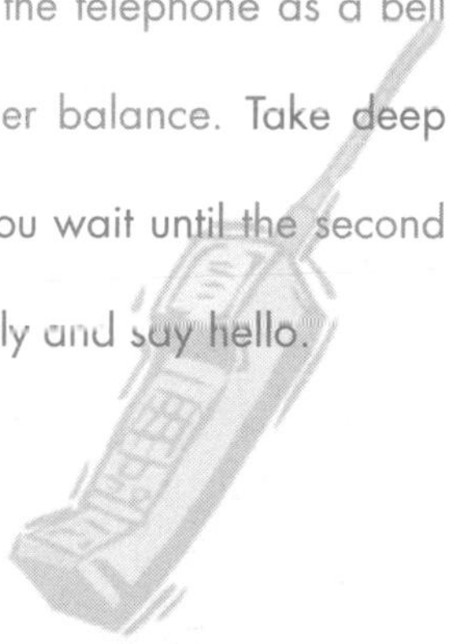

Outdoor Activity

How about ice skating, snorkeling, snow boarding, wind surfing, or horseback riding? See the world in new ways; seek wisdom in the open air. Start on the "bunny slopes" with an encouraging instructor to make it a relaxing and rewarding experience.

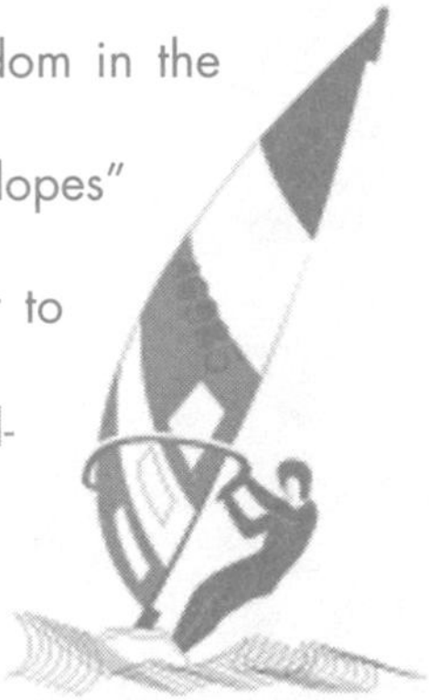

Find the Calm after the Storm

Rainbow searching is both an art and a science. The magical arc of all colors appears as a result of the refractive dispersion of sunlight. Following a rain, look in the direction opposite the sun and you just might spot the spectrum.

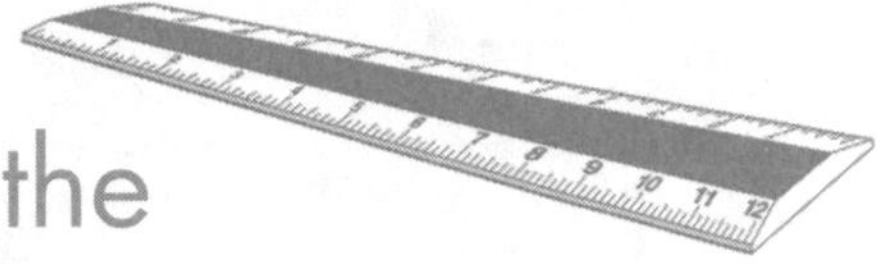

Measure the Value of Your Activities

Ask yourself, "Is this task important or urgent?" To save time for the things you really want to do, avoid unnecessary meetings, cancel unimportant commitments, screen phone calls, and limit time spent responding to e-mail and other messages.

Provide a physical **OUTLET** for anger and frustration. Don't make someone else your target — just express the feelings you are experiencing. Punch a pillow as a tool for temporary release. Then take time to plan a positive solution.

Learn to Juggle

This fun-filled challenge will unravel your jangled nerves. And clowning around also has its serious side. If you stick with it, you will develop a meditative concentration.

Go to the playground and kid around on the swings, slide, and seesaw.

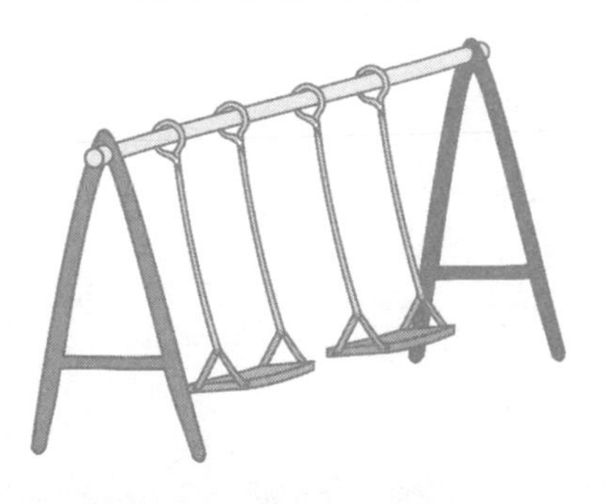

Gauge Your Stress

Chart your stress level on a scale of 1 (totally calm) to 10 (over the top) every morning and evening for a week. Increased awareness and realistic expectations will help you find solutions to lower your stress level a notch or two.

Sometimes the old standby of slowly **COUNTING** to 10 before you speak is not strong enough to soothe you. Try to subtract some of your worry time with arithmetic. When stressed, silently count backward from 100 by sevens. Your focus and concentration will add up to a more relaxed solution.

“The winds of grace
are blowing
all the time,
and it’s up to us
to raise our sails.”

Father Thomas Keating

Stand Your Ground

Protect yourself from pushy people and unreasonable requests. An aggressive stance will hurt the other person; a passive posture will harm you. But if you assertively state your personal limits, you'll feel more self-assured in a peaceful position.

Do the Opposite

One of the easiest ways to bring calm to a stressful day is to reverse your position. When you've been indoors, go outside for 5 minutes; when you are sitting at a desk, stand up; and when you have been with people, take 5 minutes alone. This technique also soothes cranky children.

Chest-Expanding Stretch

This stretch will help you breathe easier.

1. Stand up. Place your palms on your buttocks.
2. Inhale and gently raise your head while stretching your hands up and back, away from your body. Imagine that you are holding a lemon between your shoulder blades.
3. Exhale and release.

Explore
a place of
enchantment.

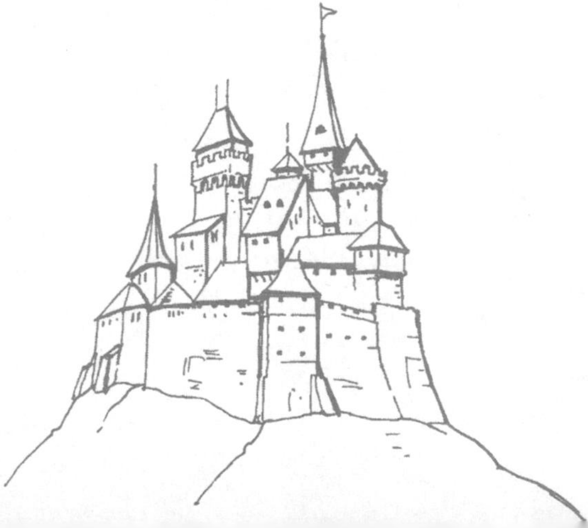

H-A-L-T

Use this 12-step-program slogan as a reminder: When Hungry, Angry, Lonely, or Tired, resist the impulse to overeat, drink alcohol, or make other choices with negative consequences. Healthier alternatives, such as a small snack or extra sleep, will calm and console you.

Collect Special Items

Bring home matchbooks from restaurants, stones and rocks with pleasing shapes, porcelain miniatures, or little decorative boxes. Choose meaningful objects that are also inexpensive, easy to clean, and easily transportable. Recollect the people and places associated with your items.

Reread an old favorite. Eliminate suspense — you already know how it ends.

Treat yourself to some **REFINED** relaxation. Take an intermission from your chores this weekend to attend a cultural event. Ask a friend to accompany you to a play, art film, ballet, or opera.

Sacred Circle

Attend a monthly meditation meeting or start a men's or women's group. Gather together with others to share sacred silence and to explore emotions.

Fortune Telling

Spend an evening with the secrets of tarot cards, runes, or the *I Ching*. These fortune-telling methods can take you on a magical tour through your inner desires. It is predicted that even those who are not serious practitioners of divination will benefit from the intuitive process.

Cool down the calorie- and caffeine-free way. A pitcher of iced herbal tea is a perfect soother on a hot summer's day. Pour yourself a tall, **CHILLED** glass of chamomile or lemon balm tea and garnish with a sprig of fresh mint.

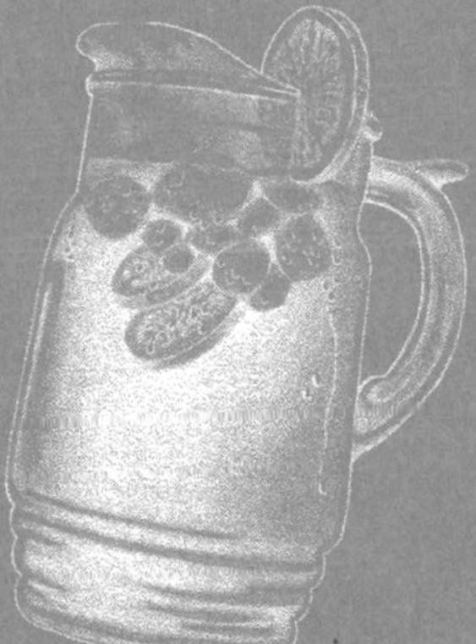

Design your own relaxation **TRAINING** period. Begin the season with 20 minutes of yoga or meditation four times a week. After three weeks, increase your sessions to 40 minutes, six days a week. In three months, you'll be a pro!

Make Peace with Your Past

Cultivating forgiveness is complex. Forgive yourself for any regrets, but don't force yourself into a resolution. Forgiveness will help you let go of guilt, anger, anxiety, and fear. Remember — you are more affected by negative feelings and memories than the other person involved.

Sweet Dreams

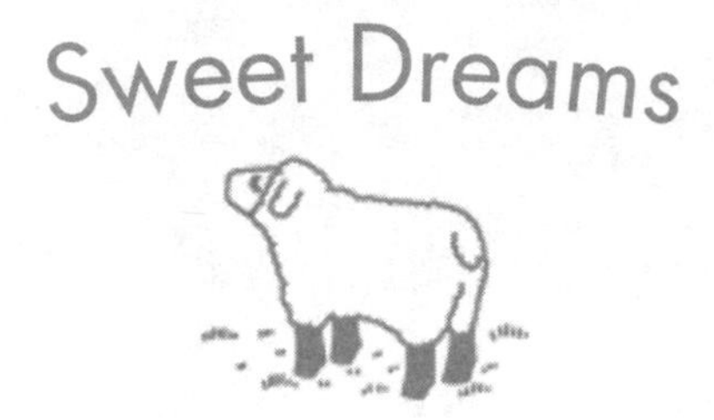

Can't sleep? Count sheep. When you visualize sheep jumping one by one over a white picket fence, you use your imagination as a sleep-enhancing ally. Focusing on a repetitive image leaves little mental brain space for worries that keep you awake.

Find Your Dream Job

When work becomes a nightmare, take time to imagine your ideal vocation. Find a supportive coach or career counselor. Take a test of your aptitudes and skills. Follow your chosen path.

"When we find our rhythm of compassion we have come home, we are in a state of grace. We are in tune with a great universal cadence where a rich inner life is exquisitely balanced with a passionate engagement with the world."

Gail Straub

Be Here Now

The first step toward relaxation is awareness. Ask yourself, "What is going on inside my body right now?" and "What is currently happening in the world around me?" First focus on physical sensations and describe your inner environment. Then observe external events and identify the sights, sounds, and smells around you. Differentiate between your inner and outer space to help you be fully present in the moment.

Treat yourself to a **SENSUAL** eye pillow. The best ones are narrow rectangles of silk or velvet filled with flaxseed and aromatic herbs. Lie down, close your eyes, and drape the pillow over your face.

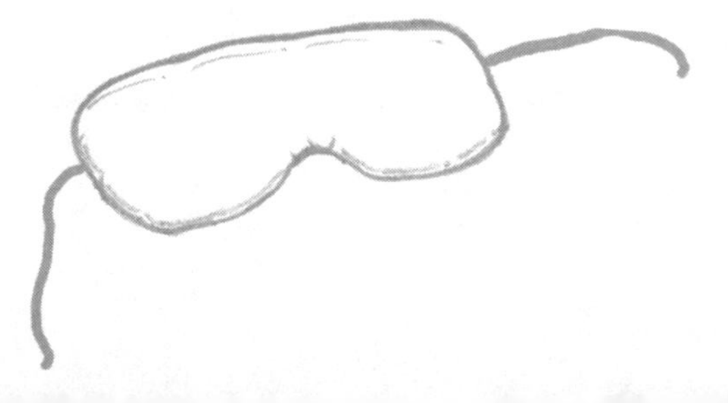

Ask for Help

Ask your friends, family, and colleagues for assistance. Of course, there is no guarantee that you will get what you want. But it's even less likely if you don't ask.

Calm Down with Chamomile

Chamomile tea, served hot or chilled, is a mild-tasting, wonderfully relaxing beverage. Sleepless adults and cranky children also benefit when dried chamomile flowers are added to an evening bath.

Grace your house with a symbol of **SERENITY.** Choose a personally meaningful image or figurine that connotes protection and blessing. Every time you cross your threshold, it will remind you to relax.

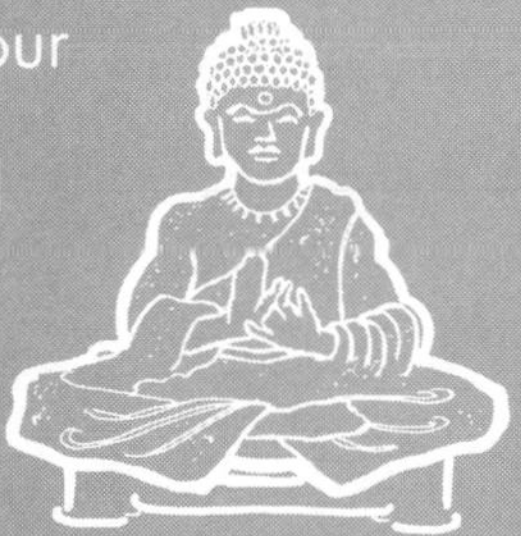

"People who have a lot of money and no time we call 'rich.' People who have time but no money we call 'poor.' Yet the most precious gifts — love, friendship, time with loved ones — grow only in the sweet soil of 'unproductive' time."

Wayne Muller

APPRECIATE your own achievements. Praise yourself when you're patient. Reward yourself for learning to relax. Honor your heartening activities. Encourage your internal intentions.

Soulful kudos to you. . .

Other Storey Titles You Will Enjoy

The Healing Aromatherapy Bath, by Margo Valentine Lazzara. This hands-on approach to mind/body healing includes aromatherapy recipes, imagery exercises, and meditation techniques for reducing stress and promoting sound sleep. 144 pages. Paperback. ISBN 1-58017-197-4.

Rosemary Gladstar's Herbs for Reducing Stress & Anxiety, by Rosemary Gladstar. One of America's foremost herbalists provides practical information for using herbs to reverse the damage of daily stress and strengthen the nervous system. 80 pages. Paperback. ISBN 1-58017-155-9.

365 Ways to Energize Mind, Body & Soul, by Stephanie Tourles. This fun-to-read gift book offers 365 simple, effective ways to increase your energy and vitality. 384 pages. Paperback. ISBN 1-58017-331-4.

These books and other Storey books are available at your bookstore, farm store, garden center, or directly from Storey Books, 210 MASS MoCA Way, North Adams, MA 01247, or by calling 800-441-5700. Or visit our Web site at www.storey.com